Peer Support Work in Mental Health Services

Responding to a growing understanding surrounding the unique knowledge and skill set of individuals with lived experience of mental health conditions, this book fills a gap in current literature by exploring the role of peer support work through the four realms of theory, research, policy and practice with a particular focus on mental health discourses.

Filled with practical case studies and guidance on the most effective approaches to peer support work, these chapters support readers in building their knowledge of the following:

- The theoretical models of peer work, including historical underpinnings, benefits and drawbacks, and the ontological, epistemological basis for lived experience as a knowledge sub-set.
- The research behind the value of experiential knowledge, models of peer support work, ethical dilemmas and how peer support work relates to traditional mental health discourse.
- The policy developments in relation to peer support work.
- Peer support work in practice, including work with families, support work specialisms and current guidance on best practice.

A must-read for those working within mental health services, this book provides a comprehensive guide to peer support work for mental health professionals, programme managers, peer support workers and service users.

Michael John Norton is Recovery and Engagement Programme Lead with the HSE Office of Mental Health Engagement and Recovery. One of Michael's main areas of responsibility is peer support work due to his past experiences of being a peer support worker for the HSE mental health services in the Republic of Ireland. Michael is also a lecturer at University College Cork, Ireland.

'In this important book, Michael John Norton draws together his deep experience and national leadership of mental health peer support work in Ireland. He skilfully takes the reader on a journey, describing how peer support work is part of a wider mental health system transformation. I was particularly impressed by his thoughtful discussion of lived experience, the ethical and implementation challenges created by peer support work, and his insights on working with specific groups, e.g. families, young people and forensic populations. This book will influence policy and practice, both within and beyond Ireland.'

Mike Slade, *Professor of Mental Health Recovery and Social Inclusion, University of Nottingham, UK*

'*Peer Support Work in Mental Health Services: Theory, Research, Policy and Practice* provides a unique synthesis of evidence, policy and practice from the standpoint of lived experience. The author brings extensive experiential wisdom from multiple sources: as someone who uses mental health services, has been employed as a peer support worker, has led the implementation of peer support across Ireland and is an academic, working in university education and research. Norton distils information from various sources (people, places, practice, theories, policies and research) to provide a comprehensive critical analysis and interpretation of the current position of peer support. This is enriched by relevant and accessible case studies from experienced peer workers with specific expertise. Norton not only explores the conflicts, dilemmas and questions that surround peer support, he also draws on evidence to construct new models for understanding the role and mechanisms underpinning peer support, and to pose resolutions and topics for further research. This is an invaluable text for anyone working as a peer support worker and for those planning, managing or seeking to understand the potential of peer support and lived experience as an essential contributor to system transformation.'

Julie Repper, *CEO, ImROC*

'I think this new book on intentional peer support working in mental health services richly adds to the discourse on peer support working and the understanding of the work. It explores the development of peer support working as an intentional and professional application of lived experience and gives some very important and insightful understanding to the development of peer support working. In that regard the book sets out useful definitions of both 'Peer support working' and 'Lived experience'. There is also a very useful discussion contained in the book around the ethical challenges of issues including the role of mutuality and reciprocity and how they are actualised in intentional peer support. Overall the book is a welcome addition to the repository of knowledge on Peer support working in services based on a review of the practical experience of developments in recent decades as well as the author's own insights. It will be of benefit to people interested in peer support working and to services wishing to introduce and improve peer support working. And most importantly I think it provides a platform for further enriched discussion and advances in peer support working in the coming years by providing a base line of current practice and understandings of the role.'

Michael Ryan, *Head of the Office of Mental Health Engagement and Recovery, Republic of Ireland*

Peer Support Work in Mental Health Services

Theory, Research, Policy and Practice

Michael John Norton

Routledge
Taylor & Francis Group

LONDON AND NEW YORK

First published 2026
by Routledge
4 Park Square, Milton Park, Abingdon, Oxon OX14 4RN

and by Routledge
605 Third Avenue, New York, NY 10158

Routledge is an imprint of the Taylor & Francis Group, an informa business

© 2026 Michael John Norton

British Library Cataloguing-in-Publication Data
A catalogue record for this book is available from the British Library

ISBN: 978-1-032-71704-3 (hbk)
ISBN: 978-1-032-71453-0 pbk)
ISBN: 978-1-032-71705-0 (ebk)

DOI: 10.4324/9781032717050

Typeset in Times New Roman
by Newgen Publishing UK

Contents

Figures

Tables

Case Study Contributors

Karen Beveridge is an educator and advocate who has faced and overcome challenges. She uses her personal experiences and knowledge to produce and co-produce a variety of courses and workshops. With a background in delivering and assessing health and social care courses, she offers a unique and valuable perspective when facilitating. She is a passionate believer in the power of education to bring about positive change in people's lives and is deeply committed to using her experiences to support and uplift others.

Racheal Burns (she/her) is a 21-year-old Western Australian with a passion for youth mental health and disability advocacy. She has a wealth of lived experience alongside a thirst for knowledge, a drive for justice and a passion for humanity. She hopes to make lasting and meaningful changes on both individual and systemic levels.

Nina Eck, MSW, was the first peer hired at the psychiatric departments of Iceland's National University Hospital in 2021. Since then, she has become a trainer with Intentional Peer Support Iceland and worked on implementing peer support into more of the hospital's departments. Nina identifies as Mad and has focused on destigmatisation of mental illness, advocating for user involvement and right to self-determination. She graduated as a social worker in 2024 and wrote her thesis on health care professionals' experience of peer support implementation.

William Gallini-Poole is a senior peer specialist as well as a coordinator for neurodiversity down in Dorset. He specialises in neurodiversity and young persons' work while also helping with inclusion. He has been working in lived experience for five years and volunteering for another three.

Matthew Jackman identifies as a Mad person. They received Australia's National Mental Health Advocate award from the Mental Health Foundation of Australia in 2020. Matthew is Founder/Principle Consultant of The Australian Centre for Lived Experience, an international peer-led consultancy and advisory practice. They have been a global mental health activist promoting human rights, social justice and lived experience perspective from public health, critical sociology and Mad studies disciplines. Matthew's advocacy career addresses alternatives to the biological, psychiatric and 'psy' science approaches to wellbeing, with a focus on social, cultural, spiritual and structural determinants. Matthew previously represented the Western Pacific Region on the Global Mental Health Peer Network and was Global Shaper with the World Economic Forum. They consult the World Health Organisation on lived experience, mental health perspective and peer work practice. Matthew trained locally in undergraduate and postgraduate social work. Furthermore, they trained internationally in certified peer specialist practice at Project Return in Los Angeles. They have been a social work lecturer in mental health and trauma for a decade. Matthew has been a long-standing public servant in forensic mental health, the Department of Social Services, and the National Disability Insurance Agency. Matthew is an open service user, participant, consumer and family/carer of various systems. They are passionate about dismantling and reconstructing systems of justice-driven care. Matthew is currently undertaking their PhD at the University of Sydney under Professor Jennifer Smith Merry and Professor Brendan McCormack investigating the influence of Mad studies as a theoretical and philosophical foundational underpinning to the consumer/survivor/user/ex-patient/Mad movement.

Lydia Little is a neurodivergent practitioner-manager and doctoral researcher specialising in psychological trauma, with a focus on the lived experiences of professionals in health and social care. Her research explores the identity paradox of being both patient and professional, as well as the role of value-based practice in peer work. After several years overseeing peer mental health services in the third sector, she now leads services for a major domestic abuse charity in Southwest UK. She is committed to recognising the unique strengths and skills that staff with lived experience bring to caring professions.

Sandra O'Sullivan is a support practitioner working in Stirling, Scotland with the Richmond Fellowship. She studied peer support working in mental health at Dublin City University in 2022–2023. She moved to Scotland where she studied Mental Health Awareness at North East College, Scotland. She hopes to continue her studies in Trauma Informed Care in the future. She loves Ireland, but Scotland is now home. Edinburgh is her favourite city and she spends her spare time visiting local heritage sites. She enjoys having odd gin and lemonade and loves the sea. She has a great love of music and dogs but her favourite animal is the highland COO.

Nicole Troy's personal background with mental health difficulties began when she struggled as a teenager experiencing extreme bouts of anxiety, an eating disorder, self-harm and suicidal ideation. In addition, Nicole also grew up in a loving family and was also raised by a parent with various mental health diagnoses. Nicole's teenage years inspired her to help others with similar circumstances and backgrounds. Nicole's own mental health issues enabled and equipped her to understand both herself and others, as well as develop empathy and patience for herself and those who have had and who are going through similar experiences. Nicole stated that, most importantly, her issues inspired her to promote recovery and instil hope in others as often as possible in every interaction she would have. As a result of Nicole's various stents of therapy throughout her teenage years, she began to realise and recognise that experiencing any of the above struggles does not make her any less of an individual than those who do not experience mental health difficulties. Instead, her struggles inspired her to research and understand the depth of despair that many people face at any time, and at any stage in life. Mental health is health, and no one is immune. Over time through various psychology modules in her BA and further through her research and studies during her MSc, Nicole began to research, develop and investigate preferences for her own coping skills through various bouts of trial and error, research and support from others. She began using various coping strategies, affirmations, reflective writings and other wellbeing methods to support herself while struggling. One of her main thoughts during this period, and that still reflects on today, was 'If I can do this once, I can do it all again.' With each step back, she learns something more about herself and utilises it for future experiences. Something sparked resilience within Nicole, and within her recovery journey, she took one day at a time.

Olga Zilberberg is a trained CBT and NLP practitioner specialising in Neuro-Affirming practices and Positive Mental Health. She has been working with charities, the voluntary sector, councils and Mental Health Recovery Colleges across the country for the past decade. Her devotion to mental health recovery and education stems from her own personal challenges in her mid-20s, driving her commitment to supporting others on their recovery journeys. With extensive experience working in Recovery Colleges, Olga has trained staff members in 14 colleges nationwide on incorporating neuro-affirming practices into recovery education. She skilfully combines her firsthand experiences with her academic expertise to empower individuals and foster positive change in their lives. Olga's mission is to share her knowledge through co-produced workshops, helping people lead happier, more fulfilling lives. Her dedication to bridging the gap between traditional mental health programmes and neurodiversity inclusion is rooted in her personal journey advocating for her neurodivergent children. These experiences have ignited her desire to champion neurodiversity awareness, inclusion and understanding in society. In addition to her professional work, Olga volunteers with Neurodiversity in Business, where she delivers neurodiversity awareness sessions to corporate members. Since joining the charity in 2022, she has passionately contributed to their mission of fostering inclusive environments where every individual can thrive.

Preface

This book marks the third text I have created in the past three years. This time, the subject is something I have given all my life in recovery trying to understand and, in a way, perfect. When I first began my recovery journey in 2015, I was first introduced to peer support work by a nurse who worked in the local day services: Fiona. Fiona and I became great friends over the years, but I will always remember being introduced to this way of working by her, as for the first time, I did not have to hide who I really was. My experiences were of importance and could be used to support others so that no one else would have to walk that journey on their own ever again.

In Ireland, the role of the Peer Support Worker was rolled out by statutory mental health services in 2017 and I was one of the first 30 statutory peers working for the services. I remember the training was simple but, at the same time, complex. We spoke about community and the therapeutic application of lived experience as well as how peers are situated within traditional mental health discourse. My first team was an older adult team where I found that although the people, I was working with, were easily 50 years older than me, I could still connect with them on a subconscious level through our shared experiences. Here I first began to explore a space that would become informality as a form of therapeutic space that can support pure mutuality, reciprocity and connection. Indeed, this enquiry led me to later publish a letter to the editor of the *Irish Journal of Psychological Medicine* entitled "*More than Just A Health Care Assistant: Peer Support Working within Rehabilitation and Recovery Mental Health Services.*" This publication was the first to name informality outright as a space that's therapeutic within peer support work. However, this article was also influenced by a master's research that I was conducting at that time into peer support work in mental health.

In April 2020, at the height of the COVID-19 pandemic, I progressed into a new role within statutory services where I would become the national lead for the peer support initiative in an Irish context. I remained dedicated to this role until late last year (September 2024) when I officially commenced a PhD. During my tenure in this post, I wrote excessively about peer support working, recovery and experiential knowledge. However, it was always my dream to write a book, but the rationale for writing it only became apparent through my national lead role, when I found that, despite the literature base into peer support work, local managers and other multi-disciplinary team staff had no idea as to what the Peer Support Worker does to help an individual progress along their unique, lifelong recovery journey. As such, this text was written and constructed with this in mind.

Providing the latest evidence into the role as well as providing job descriptions, referral pathways and vignettes from case study contributors, this book allows individuals to engage with the materials they need to grasp more fully how peer support actually works at a micro-, meso- and macro level, bringing the ethos of lived experiences to the heart of mental health care conversations. It is hoped that this text will also help convince service managers to invest in the recovery paradigm and in peer support work so that those they care for and serve can be given the best possible chance of living a life of their own choosing.

Acknowledgements

This book is the third text that I have written in the past three years about the personal recovery journey and the factors that influence it. From co-production to recovery to peer support work, each of these has a special affinity for me as a scholar and as a human being, as I have experienced all three during my 33 years on this Earth. However, I am acutely aware that I would not be here without the constant support of certain individuals in my life. Firstly, to my parents, Mary Ann and John, thank you for giving me the space to excel in this field and listening to me on days when I felt like giving up. Without your continuous love and support, I am sure that I would not be alive today to achieve all that I have done in ten years since my recovery began. To my brothers, Patrick and Edward, although you do wonder what I do and how I spend all my days in front of a computer, you still are a source of support that has enhanced my recovery journey to this day, thank you. To my sister-in-law Louise, thank you for always having my back and being the elder sister I never expected to have. Thank you for bringing brightness to our family in the midst of darkness and for keeping Paddy in line. To my gorgeous goddaughter Sophie and godson Cody, I hope this book becomes a reminder that everything is possible if you set your mind to it and work hard. I hope that neither of you ever ends up in a situation where you require professional peer support, but if you do, know that although simplistic, peer support work has a science and complexity to it that is worth investing time and energy in. To my godchildren, thank you for being a source of laughter and pride as I see you both living your lives to the fullest. To my best friends Dwayne, Linda and your partner Eddie, thank you for having the patience to put up with me as a friend. I know I do not text a lot or am available a lot to do the things we love, but thank you for realising that this endeavour is important to me and for taking this into consideration when planning hangouts. Finally, this book is dedicated to the Peer Support Workers and Family Peer Support Workers of the Irish mental health services – both of those on active duty and those who have moved on from their post. This role and everything it entails would not be possible without your resilience and determination to ensure that the recovery paradigm reaches the door of every service user within the mental health service. I appreciate your continuous efforts and services to those who are in dark place, along with being the inspiration for this book.

Part 1

Introduction

Chapter 1

Context

Setting the Scene

1.1 Introduction

Peer support work is not a new concept within mental health discourse (Health Service Executive, 2020). It has been around in a multitude of forms for over a century now (see Chapter 2 for further details). However, in today's mental health services, peer support plays a pivotal role and is used to support and enhance a person's personal recovery journey from mental health difficulties (Wall et al., 2022). Despite the obvious advantages of such a role within traditional mental health service provision, challenges remain (Glynn, 2023). Such challenges (as described further in Chapter 5) are both internal and external in nature, compounded by a multitude of factors, including the lack of a clear, comprehensive and universal definition (Janouskova et al., 2022), to that of organisational culture (Kuek et al., 2021; Ramesh et al., 2023) and a complete lack of role clarity (Hunt and Byrne, 2019; Kane et al., 2023). Such challenges, as we will later see, have, over time, led to a huge exodus of those in the role to other ventures that are less stressful, with more career prospects and, ultimately, more respect for the work that they do.

As a result, this book is an attempt to address many of these salient issues, so that services – particularly management and supervisors – have a clearer understanding of the unique role. In so doing, the text will act as a catalyst for changes within the system to occur so that the lived experience of workforce can be fully embraced by traditional services. This will occur due to both the text layout and the use of vignettes throughout the text to demonstrate some aspects of peer support not only on a theoretical basis, but also in a practical light.

Part 1 comprises an introduction to this text. Part 2 examines the theoretical components of peer support work in mental health. Starting off with the historical context of the traditional mental health system itself followed by that of peer support work. Next, the possible definitions of peer support will be explored, followed by its various principles and roles. This section concludes with a critical discussion of the advantages and challenges of peer support work within traditional mental health systems. Part 3 examines the current research activities taking place within this space. For example, Chapter 6 explores the knowledge set used by peers. This is followed by an exploration of the various models of peer support

DOI: 10.4324/9781032717050-2

and the associated ethical dilemmas of peer support work. Finally, there will be a discussion on whether peer support should be placed within traditional mental health structures. Part 4 then explores mental health policy and its relationship with peer support. Part 5 examines the various practices of peer support work in mental health, including current practices and family peer support, followed by a multitude of peer support specialisms that are being developed to fully harness this resource. The final part (Part 6) concludes the text by providing a synopsis of what has been discussed whilst also providing recommendations for the future development of peer support work in mental health systems.

This chapter begins by providing the reader with some background context into peer support work in mental health service provision. Section 1.2 begins this process by exploring the global state of peer support work in mental health. This includes the current numbers of peer support staff in Ireland and internationally at the time of writing. This is then followed by Section 1.3, which discusses the growing evidence base of peer support work in mental health, concluding with a disclaimer as per the lifecycle of this text as a result of the rapid growth of evidence in this area of scholarship. Section 1.4 discusses the purpose of this text, particularly as it relates to the target audience and the rationale for same, as well as the four-pronged approach used to examine peer support work in mental health in this text and the rationale for the use of this approach. Section 1.5 concludes this chapter.

1.2 Current Global State of Peer Support Work in Mental Health

Since the 1990s, the employment of peer support workers has been recommended by both international and national mental health policies, resulting in the role now in situ in a number countries (Kotera et al., 2023). Since then, a considerable amount of work has been undertaken to implement the role in traditional service provision (Norton et al., 2023). Within an Irish context, this work first came into focus by the mental health policy document *A Vision for Change: Report of the Expert Group on Mental Health Policy* (Department of Health, 2006). This policy advocated for the dissolution of the traditional asylums of the time, the creation of multidisciplinary community mental health teams, the introduction of personal recovery as an empirical concept and the promotion of peer support practices (Department of Health, 2006; Hunt and Byrne, 2019; Norton 2022). Although there are critics of the report, it did act as a catalyst for systemic change, which resulted in the then Advancing Recovery in Ireland (ARI) publishing a guidance document to support services to begin work on service readiness for peer support workers (Naughton et al., 2015). This led in 2017 to the employment of peer support workers and later family peer support workers. In recent years, there has been a depletion of peer roles due to a number of factors, including service readiness and lack of career progression. Today, 22 peer support workers and 10 family peers are employed by or seconded to traditional services to provide experiential supports to those who are in an earlier phase of their recovery journey (Norton et al., 2023a). Figure 1.1 depicts

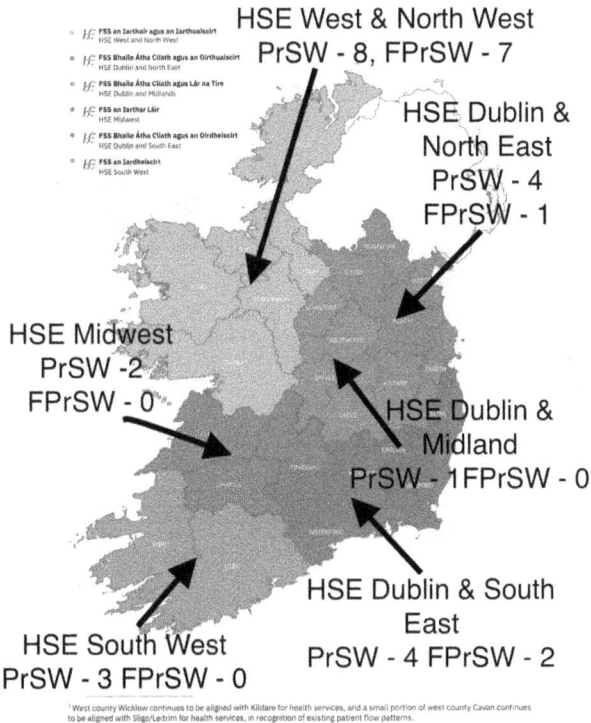

FSS an Iarthair agus an Iarthuaiscirt
HSE West and North West

FSS Bhaile Átha Cliath agus an Oirthuaiscirt
HSE Dublin and North East

FSS Bhaile Átha Cliath agus Lár na Tíre
HSE Dublin and Midlands

FSS an Iarthar Láir
HSE Midwest

FSS Bhaile Átha Cliath agus an Oirdheiscirt
HSE Dublin and South East

FSS an Iardheiscirt
HSE South West

HSE West & North West
PrSW - 8, FPrSW - 7

HSE Dublin & North East
PrSW - 4 FPrSW - 1

HSE Midwest PrSW -2 FPrSW - 0

HSE Dublin & Midland PrSW - 1FPrSW - 0

HSE Dublin & South East PrSW - 4 FPrSW - 2

HSE South West PrSW - 3 FPrSW - 0

¹ West county Wicklow continues to be aligned with Kildare for health services, and a small portion of west county Cavan continues to be aligned with Sligo/Leitrim for health services, in recognition of existing patient flow patterns.

Figure 1.1 Map of Peer and Family Peer Support Workers in Ireland.
Source: Department of Health

the placement of both peer support workers and family peer support workers in the Republic of Ireland (accurate as per date of manuscript submission).

Outside Ireland, the number of peer support workers employed by traditional statutory services is more difficult to ascertain, with many reporting outdated data. For instance, the NHS in England alone employed 742 peer support workers as of 30 September 2019 (NHS Health Education England, 2020). Additionally, as of 2016, Scotland had 80 paid peer support workers in situ, with a reported far higher number taking up unpaid peer roles (Christie, 2016). During the same time period, Wales had 381 peer leaders within their services (Mind CYMRU, n.d.), but it is important to note that the data does not differentiate whether these peer leaders were NHS-based or based within the voluntary sector. In other health services, more up-to-date data is presented. Take for instance the USA, whose current workforce figures suggest that across the country, over 30,000 peer support workers are employed in a variety of services to support individuals with their mental health, with this figure continuing to grow due to growing demand for services based on experiential knowledge (Mental Health America, 2024). The breakdown of peer support workers (called peer specialists in America) per state is illustrated in Figure 1.2a and b, which is based on a status report document from Peer Recovery (2024).

(a)

Number of Certified Peer Support Specialists Per 100,000 State/Territory/District Population

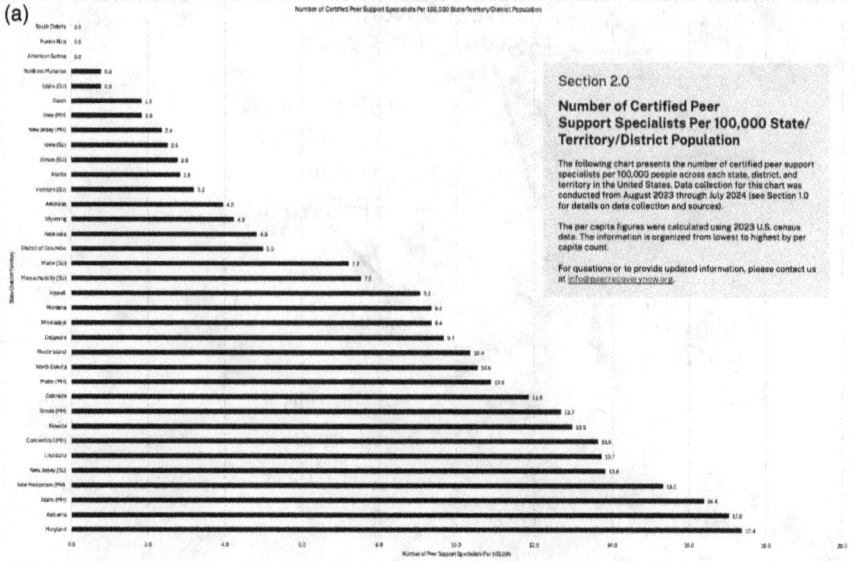

Section 2.0

Number of Certified Peer Support Specialists Per 100,000 State/ Territory/District Population

The following chart presents the number of certified peer support specialists per 100,000 people across each state, district, and territory in the United States. Data collection for this chart was conducted from August 2023 through July 2024 (see Section 1.0 for details on data collection and sources).

The per capita figures were calculated using 2023 U.S. census data. The information is organized from lowest to highest by per capita count.

For questions or to provide updated information, please contact us at info@peerrecoverynow.org.

Figure 1.2a Breakdown of Peer Specialists per State: Part One.

(b)

Number of Certified Peer Support Specialists Per 100,000 State/Territory/District Population

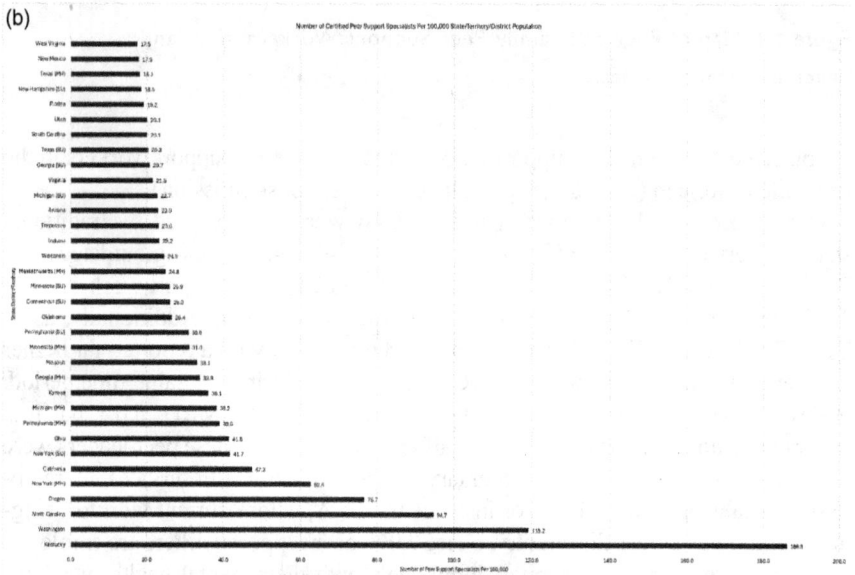

Figure 1.2b Breakdown of Peer Specialists per State: Part Two.

However, like the Welsh data, the figures presented for America do not reveal the position of these peers either within or external to the traditional health-care system. Australia reports their data differently than other jurisdictions, using a rate per 10,000 mental health care staff. In 2021/22, there were 156 peer support workers and 113 family peers per 10,000 mental health care staff in the New South Wales jurisdiction, with this figure steadily rising (Mental Health Commission of New South Wales, 2024) (see Figure 1.3a and b).

Finally, within the wider Australian states, once again there is little reliable data available. However, the figures suggest that for 2021/22 there were in excess of 360 paid peer support workers and 158 paid family peers in situ across wider Australia (Australian Government, 2024). In essence, despite the lack of reliable quantitative data relating to the state of the workforce internationally, peer support, as we will later uncover, is growing in popularity and beginning to specialise into other niche areas of mental health, including the Traveller/Roma community, other ethnic minorities, refugees and homelessness services, amongst others (Mahon, 2024).

1.3 The Evidence Base for Peer Support Work in Mental Health

Peer support is an established intervention that forms part of the broader personal recovery agenda in mental health discourse (Puschner et al., 2019). In fact,

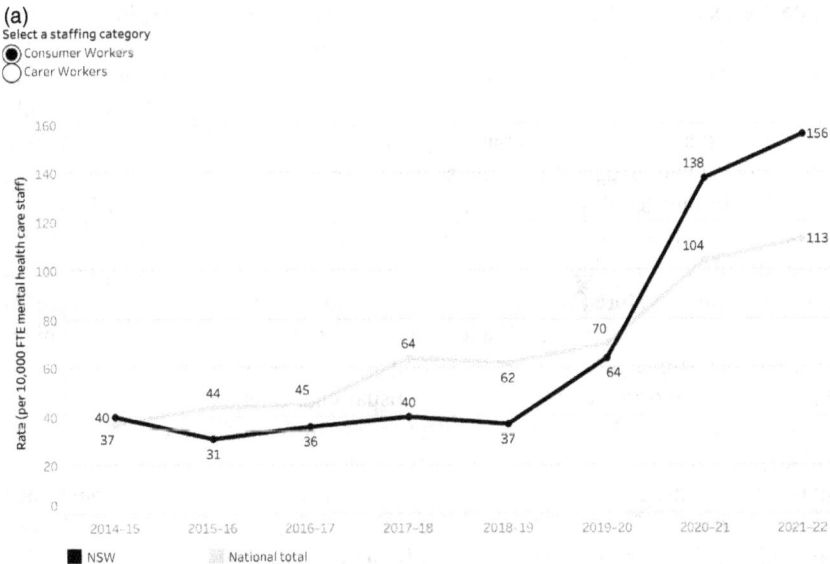

Figure 1.3a New South Wales Peer Support Workers per 10,000 Mental Health Staff.

(b)

Select a staffing category
○ Consumer Workers
◉ Carer Workers

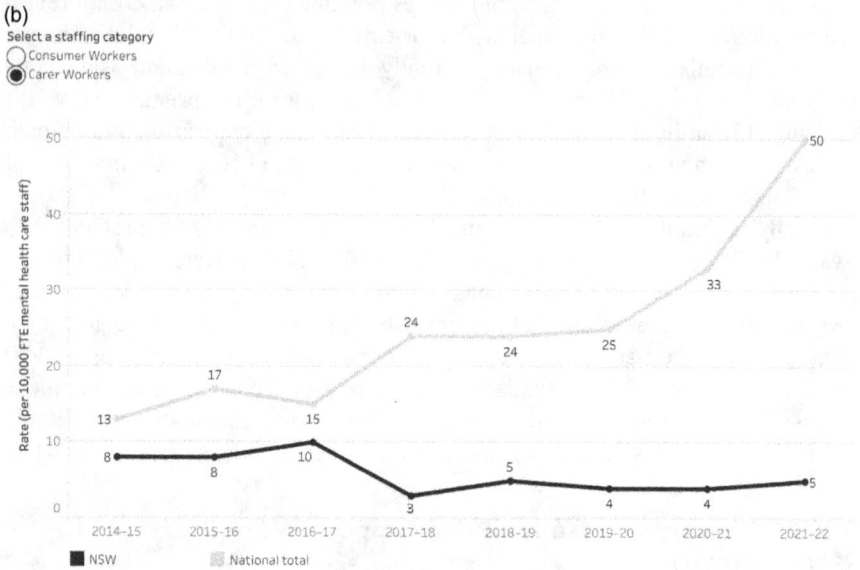

Figure 1.3b New South Wales Family Peer Support Workers per 10,000 Mental Health Staff.

despite the existence of peer support for several centuries now (explored further in Chapter 2), it is only in recent decades that the true impact of such services has been realised (Shalaby and Agyapong, 2020). This is as a result of an ever-growing evidence base for the intervention within mental health settings (Bellamy et al., 2017). For instance, in the year spanning May 2024–April 2025 alone, to the best of the author's knowledge, this is the second book to be published in this area of scholarship in the Republic of Ireland alone. Despite the growing empiricism for the concept and role, the evidence in terms of effectiveness remains unclear and indeed mixed, with findings that often contradict each other becoming common place within the literature (Wall et al., 2022; Simmons et al., 2023). For instance, in a randomised controlled trial by Steve Gillard and colleagues in 2022, they found that when one-to-one peer support was compared to that of usual care alone, peer support did not end up superior to that of usual care after 12 months post intervention. White et al. (2020) findings differ to that of Gillard and colleagues' randomised trial in that they found some areas in which peer support work excelled usual care – in this case, the greatest effect was noted on psychosocial outcomes with no significant effect noted on service user's clinical-based outcomes. Cooper et al. (2024) further contradict the work of both White et al. and Gillard et al., who identified through an umbrella review of systematic reviews that peer support is effective on some clinical outcomes as well as in terms of self-efficacy and person-led recovery outcomes.

As a result, based on the plethora of reviews available in the literature thus far, there is an increasing evidence to suggest a potential for peer support to have a positive impact on recovery-based outcomes; however, more depth into the particulars of the peer intervention is required to strengthen these claims (Murphy et al., 2023). In addition to this, the level of evidence that exists and the rate of publications that are forthcoming in relation to the concept/role means that the life-cycle of this particular text is possibly small, leading to the information provided herein being out of date relatively quickly. However, this book is necessary to help managers and supervisors in mental health to further understand the role so that they can be as supportive as possible to the various mechanisms of action for peer support. As a result, this text meets a need that services require now in order for peer support to grow and flourish in such settings.

1.4 Purpose of Present Text

Whilst the evidence base for peer support work is establishing itself, as noted in Section 1.3, the implementation of the role remains an ongoing challenge for all parties involved (Ibrahim et al., 2020). There are a number of reasons for this, including the role's impact on non-peer staff, their working conditions and confusion regarding what exactly is the role of the peer in practice within a mental health context (Shepardson et al., 2019; Haun et al., 2024). As such, this text aims to address such confusion in the literature and in practice through the use of a four-pronged approach – theory, research, policy and practice – through the fusion of theoretical concepts, the latest research along with policy integration and practical examples to demonstrate to the reader how peer support and its functions are carried out in practice. In this way, it gives the reader insight into the theoretical knowledge base behind the act whilst also demonstrating how a peer actions their role in their practice. For example, how they prepare to share the narrative, what it looks like in practice and so on. It is then hoped that with this increased understanding comes greater inter-organisational support for the peer on the ground, thus lowering the risk of another mass exodus of peers, which is currently evident in the Irish mental health service, from happening again. For example, when Hunt and Byrne published their report in 2019, there were a total of 26 peers in situ. Today, at the time of writing, there are 22 peers with more seriously contemplating leaving the role due to the above factors and also due to the pure bureaucracy and hierarchy evident within the current system.

1.5 Concluding Remarks

The purpose of this chapter was to introduce the text to the reader. It achieved this by firstly exploring the global state of peer support work in mental health. Here, we learned that peer support roles are increasing in many jurisdictions; however, gathering a definitive figure as to the amount of peer workers in any given jurisdiction is challenging due to poor record keeping on this specific issue. Despite this, from the evidence we have accumulated, one can suggest that peer support as a discipline is growing within mental health services. Added to this, we also explored the current evidence base for peer support. We identified that there are contradictions in terms of the evidence base. Some suggest that it does work, others disagree. In addition, the literature base ranges in quality from randomised controlled trials to qualitative studies to literature reviews and umbrella reviews of systematic reviews. Once this was established, the purpose of the text was discussed, specifically its focus on managers and supervisors within mental health services that may be assigned such peers in the future. Additionally, we learned how this text also serves to fill a gap in the evidence so far – the integration of the theory of peer support with practical examples of elements of peer support in action. The hope of this is that if clinicians and managers understand the complexity of peer support along with its practical application, then more supportive mechanisms will be put in place to support these very services in the retention of peer staff moving forward into the future.

References

Australian Government (2024) *Mental Health Workforce*. (Internet) Available at: www. aihw.gov.au/mental-health/topic-areas/workforce (accessed 28 July 2024).

Bellamy, C., Schmutte, T. & Davidson, L. (2017) An update on the growing evidence base for peer support. *Mental Health and Social Inclusion* 21(3), 161–167. https://doi.org/ 10.1108/MHSI-03-2017-0014

Christie, L. (2016) *Peer Support Roles in Mental Health Services*. (Internet) Available at: www.iriss.org.uk/sites/default/files/2016-06/insights-31.pdf (accessed 28 July 2024).

Cooper, R.E., Saunders, K.R.K., Greenburgh, A., Shah, P., Appleton, R., Machin, K., Jeynes, T., Barnett, P., Allan, S.M., Griffiths, J., Stuart, R., Mitchell, L., Chipp, B., Jeffreys, S., Lloyd-Evans, B., Simpson, A. & Johnson, S. (2024) The effectiveness, implementation, and experiences of peer support approaches for mental health: A systematic umbrella review. *BMC Medicine* 22, 72. https://doi.org/10.1186/s12916-024-03260-y

Department of Health (2006) *A Vision for Change: Report of the Expert Group on Mental Health Policy*. (Internet) Available at: www.hse.ie/eng/services/publications/mentalhea lth/mental-health---a-vision-for-change.pdf (accessed 28 July 2024).

Gillard, S., Bremner, S., Patel, A., Goldsmith, L., Marks, J., Foster, R., Morshead, R., White, S., Gibson, S.L., Healey, A., Lucock, M., Patel, S., Repper, J., Rinaldi, M., Simpson, A., Ussher, M., Worner, J., Priebe, S. & ENRICH Trail Study Group (2022) Peer support for discharge from inpatient mental health care versus care as usual in England (ENRICH): A parallel two-group, individually randomised controlled trial. *Lancet Psychiatry* 9, 125–136. https://doi10.1016/S2215-0366(21)00398-9

Glynn, C. (2023) *The Battle of the Peer*. (Internet) Available at: https://madinireland.com/ 2023/05/the-battle-of-the-pee (accessed 26 July 2024).

Haun, M.H., Girit, S., Goldfarb, Y., Kalha, J., Korde, P., Kwebiiha, E., Moran, G., Mtei, R., Niwemuhwezi, J., Nixdorf, R., Nugent, L., Puschner, B., Ramesh, M., Ryan, G.K., Slade, M., Charles, A. & Krumm, S. (2024) Mental health workers' perspectives on the implementation of a peer support intervention in five countries: Qualitative findings from the UPSIDES study. *BMJ Open* 14, e081962. https://doi10.1136/bmjopen-2023-081963

Health Service Executive (2020) *Peer Support Distance Working: Guidance on a Model of Peer Support Working during the Covid-19 Pandemic*. (Internet) Available at:www.hse. ie/eng/services/list/4/mental-health-services/mental-health-engagement-and-recovery/ peer-support-distance-working.pdf (accessed 26 July 2024).

Hunt, E. & Byrne, M. (2019) *Peer Support Workers in Mental Health Services: A Report on the Impact of Peer Support Workers in Mental Health Services.* (Internet) Available at: www.hse.ie/eng/services/list/4/mental-health-services/mental-health-engagem ent-and-recovery/peer-support-workers-in-mental-health-services.pdf (accessed 26 July 2024).

Ibrahim, N., Thompson, D., Nixdorf, R., Kalha, J., Mpango, R., Moran, G., Mueller-Stierlin, A., Ryan, G., Mahlke, C., Shamba, D., Puschner, B., Repper, J. & Slade, M. (2020) A systematic review of influences on implementation of peer support work for adults with mental health problems. *Social Psychiatry and Psychiatric Epidemiology* 55, 285–293. https://doi.org/10.1007/s00127-019-01739-1

Janouskova, M., Vickova, K., Harcuba, V., Kluckova, T., Motlova, J. & Motlova, L.B. (2022) The challenges of inter-role conflicts for peer support workers. *Psychiatric Services* 73(12), 1424–1427. https://doi.org/10.1176/appi.ps.202100566

Kane, L., Portman, R.M., Eberhardt, J., Walker, L., Proctor, E-L., Poulter, H. & O'Neill, C. (2023) Peer supporters' mental health and emotional wellbeing needs: Key factors and opportunities for co-produced training. *Health Expectations* 26(6), 2387–2395. https://doi.org/10.1111/hex.13836

Kotera, Y., Newby, C., Charles, A., Ng, F., Watson, E., Davidson, L., Nixdorf, R., Bradstreet, S., Brophy, L., Brasier, C., Simpson, A., Gillard, S., Puschner, B., Kidd, S.A., Mahlke, C., Sutton, A.J., Gray, L.J., Smith, E.A., Ashmore, A., Pomberth, S. & Slade, M. (2023) Typology of mental health peer support work components: Systematised review and expert consultation. *International Journal of Mental Health and Addiction.* https://doi. org/10.1007/s11469-023-01126-7

Kuek, J.H.L., Chua, H.C. & Poremski, D. (2021) Barriers and facilitators of peer support work in a large psychiatric hospital: A thematic analysis. *General Psychiatry* 34(3), e100521. https://doi10.1136/gpsych-2021-100521

Mahon, D. (2024) *Peer Support Work: Practice, Training and Implementation.* Emerald Publishing, Leeds.

Mental Health America (2024) *The Peer Workforce.* (Internet) Available at: www.mhan ational.org/peer-workforce#:~:text=Current%20workforce%20estimates%20show%20o ver,in%20which%20peers%20serve%20people (accessed 28 July 2024).

Mental Health Commission (2024) *Mental Health Consumer and Carer Peer Workers.* (Internet) Available at: www.nswmentalhealthcommission.com.au/measuring-change-indicator/mental-health-consumer-and-carer-peer-workers (accessed 28 July 2024).

Mind CYMRU (n.d.) *Peer Support in Wales: Side by Side CYMRU Improving Peer Leader Capacity to Deliver Impactful Support across Wales.* (Internet) Available at: www.mind. org.uk/media/7138/side-by-side-cymru-executive-summary-english.pdf (accessed 28 July 2024).

Murphy, R., Huggard, L., Fitzgerald, A., Hennessy, E. & Booth, A. (2023) A systematic scoping review of peer support interventions in integrated primary youth mental health care. *Journal of Community Psychology* 52(1), 154–180. https://doi.org/10.1002/jcop.23090

Naughton, L., Collins, P. & Ryan, M. (2015) *Peer Support Workers: A Guidance Paper.* (Internet) Available at: www.lenus.ie/bitstream/handle/10147/576059/PeerSupportWo rkersAGuidancePaper.pdf?sequence=6&isAllowed=y (accessed 28 July 2024).

NHS Health Education England (2020) *National Workforce Stocktake of Mental Health Peer Support Workers in NHS Trusts.* (Internet) Available at: www.hee.nhs.uk/sites/defa ult/files/documents/NHS%20Peer%20Support%20Worker%20Benchmarking%20report. pdf (accessed 28 July 2024).

Norton, M.J. (2022) More than just a health care assistant: Peer support working within rehabilitation and recovery mental health services. *Irish Journal of Psychological Medicine* 1–2. https://doi10.1017/ipm.2022.32

Norton, M.J., Clabby, P., Coyle, B., Cruickshank, J., Davidson, G., Greer, K., Kilcommins, M., McCartan, C., McGuire, E., McGilloway, S., Mulholland, C., O'Connell-Gannon, M., Pepper, D., Shannon, C., Swords, C., Walsh, J. & Webb, P. (2023) *Peer Support Work: An International Scoping Review*. (Internet) Available at: www.impactresearchcentre.co.uk/site/wp-content/uploads/2023/12/Peer-Support-Work-Scoping-Review.pdf (accessed 28 July 2024).

Norton, M.J., Griffin, M., Collins, M., Clark, M. & Browne, E. (2023a) Using autoethnography to reflect on peer support supervision in an Irish context. *Journal of Practice Teaching and Learning* 20(2). doi: https://doi.org/10.1921/jpts.v21i2.2079

Peer Recovery (2024) *National Distribution of Certified Peer Support Specialists in the United States by State district, and Territory*. (Internet) Available at: https://static1.squarespace.com/static/67017deb9fbcef5ab5aa6989/t/672d352f3901aa74aa19fa7d/1731015986795/2024-AUG-28-prcoe-numbers-report.pdf (accessed 16 August 2024).

Puschner, B., Repper, J., Mahlke, C., Nixdorf, R., Basangwa, D., Nakku, J., Ryan, G., Baillie, D., Shamba, D., Ramesh, M., Moran, G., Lachmann, M., Kalha, J., Pathare, S., Muller-Stierlin, A. & Slade, M. (2019) Using peer support in developing empowering mental health services (UPSIDES): Background, rationale and methodology. *Annals of Global Health* 85(1), 53. https://doi10.5334/aogh.2435

Ramesh, M., Charles, A., Grayzman, A., Hiltensperger, R., Kalha, J., Kulkarni, A., Mahlke, C., Moran, G.S., Mpango, R., Mueller-Stierlin, A.S., Nixdorf, R., Ryan, G.K., Shamba, D. & Slade, M. (2023) Societal and organisational influences on implementation of mental health peer support work in low-income and high-income settings: A qualitative focus group study. *BMJ Open* 13(8), e058724. https://doi 10.1136/bmjopen-2021-058724

Shalaby, R.A.H. & Agyapong, V.I.O. (2020) Peer support in mental health: Literature review. *JMIR Mental Health* 7(6), e15572. https://doi 10.2196/15572

Shepardson, R.L., Johnson, E.M., Possemato, K., Arigo, D. & Funderburk, J.S. (2019) Perceived barriers and facilitators to implementation of peer support in veterans health administration primary care-mental health integration settings. *Psychiatric Services* 16(3), 433–444. https://doi 10.1037/ser0000242

Simmons, M.B., Cartner, S., MacDonald, R., Whitson, S., Bailey, A. & Brown, E. (2023) The effectiveness of peer support from a person with lived experience of mental health challenges for young people with anxiety and depression: A systematic review. *BMC Psychiatry* 23, 194. https://doi 10.1186/s12888-023-04578-2

Wall, A., Lovheden, T., Landgren, K. & Stjernsward, S. (2022) Experiences and challenges in the role as peer support workers in a Swedish mental health context – An interview study. *Issues in Mental Health Nursing* 43(4), 344–355. https://doi 10.1080/01612840.2021.1978596

White, S., Foster, R., Marks, J., Morshead, R., Goldsmith, L., Barlow, S., Sin, J. & Gillard, S. (2020) The effectiveness of one-to-one peer support in mental health services: A systematic review and meta-analysis. *BMC Psychiatry* 20, 534. doi: https://doi.org/10.1186/s12888-020-02923-3

Part 2

Theory of Peer Support Work

Chapter 2

Historical Underpinnings of Mental Health Service Provision Inclusive of the History of the Peer Support Movement

2.1 Introduction

Mental health services have changed dramatically throughout the years. In fact, in recent years, they have changed on a structural, systemic, philosophical and cultural basis (Norton, 2021). As a result of the growing understanding, particularly in the past 150 years or so of the need for appropriate, humane services have been offered to those who present as mentally ill (Thompson, 1994). However, at the time of writing this (2024), we are still far from reaching this ideal state. There are many factors for this, including economic, political and societal perspectives of those who have a mental illness (Kelly, 2022b). The strive for the ideal mental health service in Ireland has picked up in recent years due to the publication and implementation of '*Sharing the Vision*' (Department of Health, 2020, 2022) and the reform of the '*Mental Health Act*' (Oireachtas, 2024). However, more is needed so that a service that treats each individual as a person and not a symptom of disease can become a reality.

This present chapter elaborates Chapter 1 by exploring the history of mental health service provision. Due to the complexity of mental health service provision throughout the ages, this chapter will not go, in detail, into each aspect of its history. Instead, it serves as a high-level summary to contextualise peer support as a mental health intervention to those that would have been used in the past. For a detailed examination of the history of mental health, particularly in an Irish context, see Brendan Kelly's 2019 and 2022a works. This high-level historical overview is noted in Section 2.2. Section 2.3 adds to the high-level discussions on the history of mental health service provision by discussing the historical development of peer support, from Harry Stack Sullivan to present day peer support-based activity. Section 2.4 explores multiple understandings of the causes of mental distress. This section will include an exploration of the biomedical model, stress vulnerability model and trauma, to name just a few. The chapter concludes in Section 2.5 with a summarisation followed by a brief, high-level discussion on where peer support working is moving towards internationally – particularly around the idea of peer support not being placed within the system, but instead operating external to the system.

DOI: 10.4324/9781032717050-4

2.2 A Brief History of Mental Health Service Provision

The history of mental health service provision is considered long and often dark in nature. Within the past 2 millennia, the consensus regarding the causes of mental ill health has interplayed between divine forces based on earthly elements to that of evidence and reason (Figure 2.1).

As already suggested, in this text, the purpose is not to explore the history of mental health in detail, rather to help set a context whereby one can situate the peer support movement in. In Figure 2.2, the main historical highlights of mental health are visually depicted, specifically from the 1800s onwards.

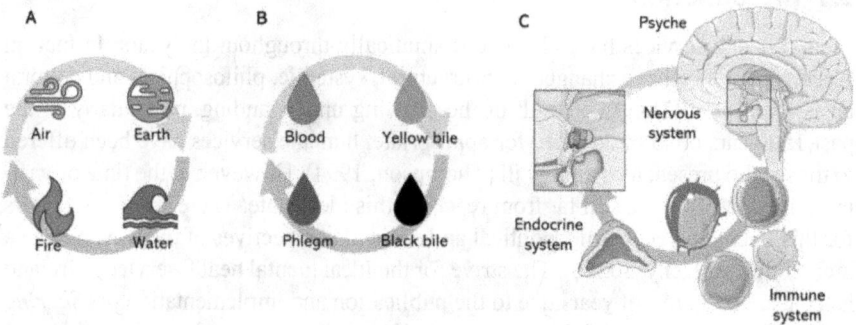

Figure 2.1 The Journey towards Evidence and Reason.

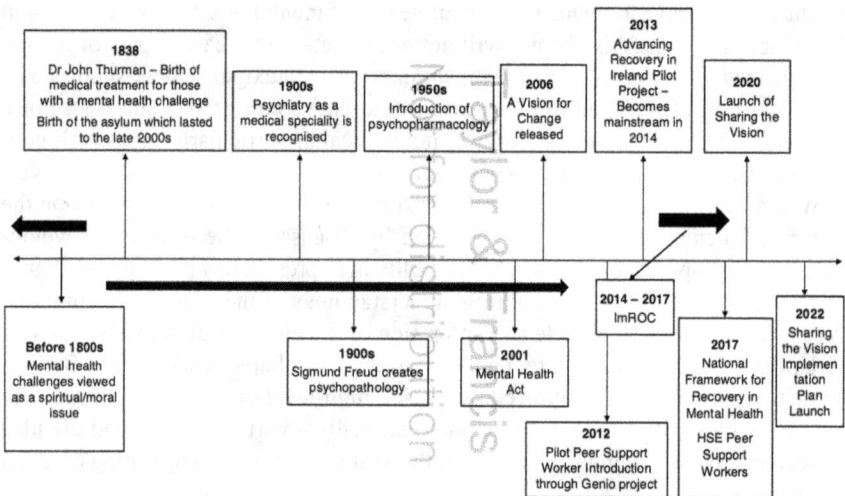

Figure 2.2 Mental Health through the Ages – A Detailed Timeline.

Since the dawn of time, scholars have longed to answer the question relating to the innermost meaning attributed to mental health challenges (Norton and Cullen, 2024). This longing is millennia old, but for the purposes of this text, we will explore from the time of Hippocrates, who first began to use evidence and reason to determine issues pertaining to health and illness. Hippocrates, who lived from 460–370 BC, is known as the father of modern medicine for his works on the theory of the four humours (Yapijakis, 2009; Lempesis et al., 2024). At this time, medicine had close ties with that of philosophy (Kalachanis and Tsagkaris, 2020). However, the development of the theory of the four humours was an attempt by Hippocrates to identify the basic constitutes of the human body which was someway scientific in nature (Kalachanis and Michailidis, 2015). Hippocrates believed that the human body was made up of four humours (blood, phlegm, yellow bile and black bile). When concentrated in the right amounts, these four elements allowed the body to remain in homeostasis (Lagay, 2002). As such, illness, including mental ill health, resulted from an imbalance of one or more of these four humours, treatments like purges and bleeding were often performed and, at that time, helped rebalance the concentration of the four humours(Dickinson, 1990; Norton, 2022). However, despite Hippocrates' works, the interplay of causation of mental distress continued between that of the divine and that of science until the mid-1800s when a psychiatrist by the name of Dr. John Thurman applied the life sciences and a positivist notion to mental distress (Dickinson, 1990).

This application of positivist notions to the subjective realities of mental illness began a somewhat downward spiral for the living conditions of the mentally ill as they began to be housed, first in work houses and then in mental asylums. The most famous of which was Bedlam, an asylum located in London, known for its deplorable living conditions and inhumane treatment of mentally ill (Arnold, 2008). As time moved from the 1800s to the 1900s, psychiatry became a branch of medicine and the dawn of the biomedical understanding of mental illness (see Section 2.4) had come (Norton, 2022). In the 1950s modern psychopharmacology commenced with the creation of the antipsychotic: chlorpromazine (Braslow and Marder, 2019). This replaced the traditional barbaric treatments conducted within the asylums until this time (Norton, 2022). However, electroconvulsive therapy remained and is still operated to this day, with some resistance within the literature in terms of whether it is truly effective or not and if it leads to undue harm to those who are treated with it (Read and Bentall, 2010; Moore, 2020; Read et al., 2020).

Around this time, the civil rights movement was commencing within America (Zunes and Laird, 2010). This movement turned out to have a massive, long-lasting impact on mental health services up until this very day. Although the movement was racially motivated, seeking equality for Black Americans (Clark, 1966), its legacy continues in others who would begin fighting for equality within other communities, including mental health. An example of this in modern day services is the rise of the Mad Pride Movement (Gerlach, 2023) and Drop the Disorder (Watson, 2017) to name just a few. Within an Irish context, the civil rights movement created a need for a strategic policy to enhance mental health service provision now and into the future. This led to the publication of '*The Psychiatric Services – Planning for the Future*' in 1984 (The Stationary Office, 1984). This document signalled the end of the traditional asylums, paving the way for recovery to occur within the community (Norton, 2022). However, the policy never gained traction for a variety of reasons and as such; services continued to operate under the asylum model until the publication of '*A Vision for Change*' in 2006 by the Irish Department of Health (Department of Health, 2006; Norton, 2019).

However, not much of the need for action expressed in '*The Psychiatric Services – Planning for the Future*', '*A Vision for Change*' went a couple of steps further and included the need for the recovery approach and the subsequent introduction of the lived experience workforce within traditional mental health service provision. The recovery approach has its foundations within the consumer/survivor movement and is best defined by William Anthony in his 1993 seminal works as:

a deeply personal, unique process of changing one's attitudes, values, feelings, goals, skills and/or roles. It is a way of living a satisfying, hopeful and contributing life even within the limitations caused by illness. Recovery involves the development of new meaning and purpose in one's life as one grows beyond the catastrophic effects of mental illness.

(Anthony, 1993. p. 21)

The closure of traditional asylums and the birth of community focussed practice came with it the need for such services to become recovery orientated. To support the achievement of recovery orientation, Irish services created a pilot project called Advancing Recovery in Ireland, or ARI for short. As part of the work of ARI, they supported Irish services to sign up to four of the ten ImROC (Implementing Recovery through Organisational Change) challenges including (1) changing the nature of day-to-day interactions, (2) co-produced learning, (3) developing recovery colleges and (4) staff well-being (Norton, 2023a). ARI remained working on these four organisational challenges until 2017, when it published its own recovery framework, which detailed four principles necessary for recovery within an Irish context. Within the document, the importance of lived experience was noted. It led Irish services in that same year to recruit the first 30 Peer Support Workers to be employed by traditional statutory mental health services. The implementation of alternative peer-led services was further supported in 2020, when '*Sharing the Vision*' – Ireland's new policy document was published (Department of Health, 2020). Here recovery is identified as an underlying principle and recommendation 74, in particular, seeks to expand peer-led services across the country (Norton, 2023b).

Today, despite the efforts of ARI and later Mental Health Engagement and Recovery (MHER), Irish services still have a long way to go to reach recovery orientation. However, a number of things are working in their favour. National mental health policy endorses the promotion of lived experience, peer services and recovery as part of its remit. A new '*National Framework for Recovery in Mental*

Health' (Health Service Executive, 2024) has been published with the commitment to develop an implementation plan to support its uptake within services. MHER, the office that replaced ARI, now has a strategic plan: '*Engaged in Recovery*' which lays out a plan to further develop the recovery objectives of peer support, recovery education and engagement (Health Service Executive, 2023). However, the introduction of Slaintecare threatens the work of MHER as services digress towards local governance rather than control from a national perspective. With this realisation, the future of recovery, of lived experience and of co-production remains uncertain as fear of a postcode lottery to determine what service is provided becomes ever more a reality.

2.3 History of the Peer Support Movement within and External to Mental Health

Peer support as a concept has been around for a very long time in a number of different contexts (Faulkner and Basset, 2012). Like the history of mental health in Section 2.1, the purpose of this enquiry is not to give a detailed history of the peer support movement. Rather, its purpose is to situate peer support into today's context whilst appreciating its grass roots and beginnings. A detailed timeline of the history of the peer support movement is supplied in Figure 2.3.

The exact era when peer support services began is highly contested within the literature. However, it is believed to have dated back more than three centuries to 18th century France when Jean Baptiste promoted peer support work through a letter to Philippe Pinel (Davidson et al., 2012; Shalaby and Agyapong, 2020; Hickney, 2022). However, after this point, peer support as a movement withdrew and entered

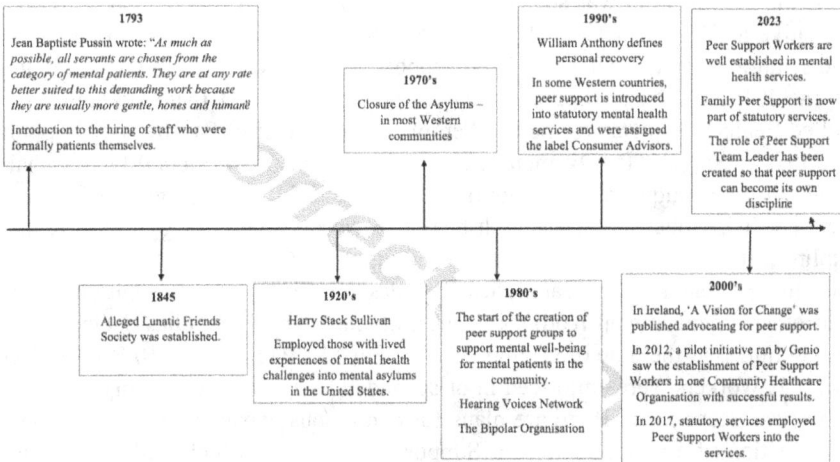

1793
Jean Baptiste Pussin wrote: "*As much as possible, all servants are chosen from the category of mental patients. They are at any rate better suited to this demanding work because they are usually more gentle, hones and humane*"

Introduction to the hiring of staff who were formally patients themselves.

1970's
Closure of the Asylums – in most Western communities

1990's
William Anthony defines personal recovery

In some Western countries, peer support is introduced into statutory mental health services and were assigned the label Consumer Advisors.

2023
Peer Support Workers are well established in mental health services.

Family Peer Support is now part of statutory services.

The role of Peer Support Team Leader has been created so that peer support can become its own discipline

1845
Alleged Lunatic Friends Society was established.

1920's
Harry Stack Sullivan

Employed those with lived experiences of mental health challenges into mental asylums in the United States.

1980's
The start of the creation of peer support groups to support mental well-being for mental patients in the community.

Hearing Voices Network

The Bipolar Organisation

2000's
In Ireland, 'A Vision for Change' was published advocating for peer support.

In 2012, a pilot initiative ran by Genio saw the establishment of Peer Support Workers in one Community Healthcare Organisation with successful results.

In 2017, statutory services employed Peer Support Workers into the services.

Figure 2.3 Peer Support within Mental Health Discourse – A Historical Timeline.

a period of regression due to the growing prominence of the biomedical understanding of mental distress (Norton, 2024). In 1845, the peer movement reattempted a resurgence through the formation of The Alleged Lunatic Friends Society – a group created to provide informal peer support to the mentally ill (Bassett et al., 2010). Since this time, peer support appeared sporadically throughout the history of mental health. In the 1920s, Harry Stack Sullivan – a psychiatrist – introduced peer support by employing former patients to support current patients recover from their mental health difficulties through the sharing and distribution of their lived experiences (Davidson et al., 2012).

In the Western world, the 1960s/70s brought a time of systemic and organisational change as the efficacy of mental asylums began to be questioned resulting in their gradual closure (Norton, 2024). This period, known as the civil rights movement, impacted those of colour as they fought for equal rights. However, it also had an impact on mental health. For instance, the movement was believed to have been a catalyst for the introduction of formalised peer support services, which is believed to have its beginnings in Georgia, United States during the 1980s (Adams, 2020). During this same time period, a number of peer support groups, like the Hearing Voices Network and The Bipolar Organisation began to emerge (Bassett et al., 2010). In the 1990s, along with the conceptualisation of recovery by Anthony (1993), the peer support movement progressed into other jurisdictions within a formal capacity, at this time under the auspices of consumer advisors (Bassett et al., 2010).

Within an Irish context, the move towards recovery and peer support began with '*A Vision for Change*' (Department of Health, 2006), when both were mentioned as an ideal within mental health service provision. This allowed for a pilot initiative by Genio to begin in 2012, in which a number of peer support positions were created in the west of Ireland to support people there with mental health difficulties. This pilot was so successful that more investment was placed on the initiative in 2016/17 to formally place Peer Support Workers under the guise of the statutory services where 30 Peer Support Workers were employed (Hunt and Byrne 2019; Norton et al., 2023). Around the same time (2015), an organisation called Bealach Nua was formed and employed a number of Family Peer Support Workers to support family members of loved ones with a mental health challenge in their unique recovery journey (Kelly, 2020) (see Chapter 12 for more details). In October 2022, the Irish health services formally recognised the discipline within traditional services by providing it with its own grade code – the first to be created in 20 years. However, despite this, due to a retention freeze and other organisational readiness issues, the number of peers has decimated in recent times. At the time of writing, 22 Peer Support Workers and 10 Family Peer Support Workers were employed in or seconded to traditional statutory services. However, despite this, there are plans for continuous expansion of the role with the creation of a new Senior Peer Support Worker role, which will have supervisory responsibility for peers in their area thus ensuring the future of the role as a self-sustaining discipline.

2.4 Various Models and Approaches to Understanding and Treating Mental Ill Health

Our understanding of mental health and mental ill health has exploded in recent years (Cullen and Norton, 2024). There are now many different models available in the literature to help us understand how someone can become mentally unwell, with many such models being contested for decades now (Richter and Dixon, 2023). However, for this text, we will focus on three such models that are prominent in mental health discourse today: the biomedical model, the stress vulnerability model and finally the trauma model. Each of them will now be explored in detail.

2.4.1 The Biomedical Model of Mental Distress

For the context of this book, the biomedical model understands mental distress as resulting from a disease of the brain relating to (1) the distribution of neurotransmitters or (2) changes in brain physiology that require pharmacological intervention to rectify these so called abnormalities (Deacon, 2013). Huda (2019) later clarifies that it is not a disease-based model. Instead, it is a pattern that is based on incorporating and comparing the clinical features of a patient to that of the known clinical features of a condition known within existing, available medical knowledge (Huda, 2019). To do this, categorical systems were created to support diagnosticians in determining a diagnosis of a particular patient with mental illness (Salicru, 2020). Such systems include the '*Diagnostic and Statistical Manual of Mental Disorders*' – DSM – developed by the American Psychiatric Association, and the '*International Classification of Diseases – Classification of Mental and Behavioural Disorders*' – ICD – developed by the World Health Organisation. Although this model has been around since the application of biology to the mentally ill, today mental health leaders are moving away from this approach towards models that are more rights based and culturally inclusive (Patel et al., 2023; Karter, 2024).

2.4.2 The Stress Vulnerability Model of Mental Distress

The stress vulnerability model originated through the work of Zubin and Spring on schizophrenia in 1977, where the model was first introduced as a rationale as to why and how a mental health challenge develops (Childs Heyl, 2023). The model accepts that there are some genetic and other biological vulnerabilities towards mental illness but asks what role stress from daily life has to play in causing a mental illness to develop (Goh and Agius, 2020). It is often depicted through the analogy of a bucket and a hose with water. The hose with water is stress, and the bucket, which has a number of holes within it, is the person. For a person who does not suffer from mental health challenges, the water from the hose goes into the bucket but then quickly escapes via the holes in the bucket, thereby maintaining homeostasis. However, if there is more water flowing into the bucket than what the holes in the bucket can handle, then the water rises to a point where it overflows from the bucket. This overflow is the person becoming overwhelmed by stress to the point that mental distress occurs. To remain mentally well, one always needs to engage in regular self-care to cope with the stress of everyday life, so that such feelings of being overwhelmed can be avoided. The stress that causes the influx of water within our analogy is created by numerous factors, including individual chronic/acute burdens, biological environment and/or the psychosocial environment (Kinser and Lyon, 2014).

2.4.3 The Trauma Model of Mental Distress

Some of the stressors noted in Section 2.4.2 may have their origins within our understanding of trauma and how this impacts the mental health of an individual. Trauma, according to Taylor and Shrive (2024), refers to any event or set of circumstances which causes severe distress and/or disturbance leading to oppression, fear, harm and/or injury. Trauma is noted as being widespread, harmful and also having an economic cost to the health services (SAMHSA's Trauma and Justice Strategic Initiative, 2014). However, how a person responds to trauma is also unique, as for one person the event or circumstance of trauma may actually have a long-lasting negative impact. For another, the event or circumstance may be completely meaningless. Regardless of how an event or circumstance of trauma may affect you, there are evidence-based links between early onset of trauma, say in childhood and the possibility of an individual attaining a serious mental disorder, like schizophrenia in their adulthood because of the trauma (Hammersley et al., 2008; Read, 2013). The trauma model is growing in popularity with many books and other sources of literature being created on the subject from authors of diverse disciplines, including psychiatry (Van Der Kolk, 2015), psychology (Read and Dillon, 2013), and psychotherapy (Mahon, 2022) (Herman, 2001). In addition, many scholars write about the idea of being trauma informed in practice leading the MHER office to co-produce a guidance document to support individual practitioners in being informed and practicing in a trauma informed manner. However, the trauma model has also received a lot of negative press for being radical in its understanding and approach leading some scholars and practitioners to dismiss it entirely (Gillis, 2024; Young, 2024). An example of this is noted within an Irish context as some two years after the guidance document's completion, but MHER has yet to formally publish it due to organisational and reputational concerns, particularly amongst the traditional disciplines.

2.5 Concluding Remarks

In summary, mental health services have changed dramatically in the last two millennia. Indeed, they are ever changing with the move today towards recovery orientation and trauma informed care. In the midst of all these changes comes the new discipline of peer support work which, for the first time, formally employed those with lived experience to support individuals with mental health difficulties in their recovery. In the short amount of time, peer support has been evident in our services, questions have already been constructed regarding peer support work and its place within the traditional system when in fact the idea of peer support is to be radical and as such radically change the way the system operates. This will be explored further in this book, but before we do so, one needs to explore peer support work further in terms of its definitions and principles so that an evidence base for peer support work is made clearly evident. The following chapters will support us on this journey by illustrating an evidence base.

References

Adams, W.E. (2020) Unintended consequences of institutionalizing peer support work in mental healthcare. *Social Science and Medicine* 262, 113249. https://doi.org/10.1016/j.socscimed.2020.113249

Anthony, W.A. (1993) Recovery from mental illness: The guiding vision of the mental health service system in the 1990s. *Psychosocial Rehabilitation Journal* 16(4), 11–23. https://doi.org/10.1037/h0095655

Arnold, C. (2008) *Bedlam: London and Its Mad.* Pocket Books, London.

Bassett, T., Faulkner, A., Repper, J. & Stamou, E. (2010) *Lived Experience Leading the Way: Peer Support in Mental Health* (Internet). Available at: https://amhp.org.uk/wp-content/uploads/2017/08/livedexperiencereport.pdf (accessed 22 September 2024).

Braslow, J.T. & Marder, S.R. (2019) History of psychopharmacology. *Annual Review of Clinical Psychology* 7(15), 25–50. https://doi.org/10.1146/annurev-clinpsy-050718-095514

Childs Heyl, J. (2023) *What Is the Stress-Vulnerability Model* (Internet). Available at: www.verywellmind.com/what-is-the-stress-vulnerability-model-history-elements-6831765 (accessed 22 September 2024).

Clark, K.B. (1966) The civil rights movement: Momentum and organization. *Daedalus* 95(1), 239–267.

Cullen, O.J. & Norton, M.J. (2024) The challenge of mental health, addiction and dual diagnosis in an Irish context. In: *Different Diagnoses, Similar Experiences: Narratives of Mental Health, Addiction Recovery and Dual Diagnosis.* (Norton, M.J & Cullen, O.J. eds.) Emerald Publishing Limited Leeds, United Kingdom. pp. 57–62.

Davidson, L., Bellamy, C., Guy, K. & Miller, R. (2012) Peer support among persons with severe mental illness: A review of evidence and experiences. *World Psychiatry* 11(2), 123–128. https://doi.org/10.1016/j.wpsyc.2012.05.009

Deacon, B.J. (2013) The biomedical model of mental disorder: A critical analysis of its validity, utility, and effect on psychotherapy research. *Clinical Psychology Review* 33(7), 846–861. https://doi.org/10.1016/j.cpr.2012.09.007

Department of Health (2006) *A Vision for Change: Report of the Expert Group on Mental Health Policy* (Internet). Available at: www.hse.ie/eng/services/publications/mentalhealth/mental-health---a-vision- for-change.pdf (accessed 08 September 2024).

Department of Health (2020) *Sharing the Vision: A Mental Health Policy for Everyone* (Internet). Available at: https://assets.gov.ie/static/documents/sharing-the-vision-a-mental-health-policy-for-everyone.pdf (Accessed 25 August 2024).

Department of Health (2022) *Implementation Plan 2022–2024: Sharing the Vision: A Mental Health Policy for Everyone* (Internet). Available at: https://assets.gov.ie/static/documents/sharing-the-vision-implementation-plan-2022-2024.pdf (accessed 25 August 2024).

Dickinson, E. (1990) From madness to mental health: A brief history of psychiatric treatments in the UK from 1800 to the present. *British Journal of Occupational Therapy* 53(10), 419–424.

Faulkner, A. & Basset, T. (2012) A long and honourable history. *The Journal of Mental Health Training, Education and Practice* 7(2), 53–59. http://dx.doi.org/10.1108/175562 21211236448

Gerlach, J. (2023) *Mad Pride and Neurodiversity – Personal Perspectives: Parallel Movements of Lived Experience* (Internet). Available at: www.psychologytoday.com/ie/blog/beyond-mental-health/202312/mad-pride-and-neurodiversity (accessed 08 September 2024).

Gillis, K. (2024) *Why Do We Dismiss Non-Physical Trauma?* (Internet) Available at: ww.psychologytoday.com/ie/blog/invisible-bruises/202404/why-do-we-dismiss-non-physical-trauma#:~:text=The%20dismissal%20of%20non%2Dphysical,of%20emo-tional%20torment%20and%20manipulation (accessed 29 September 2024).

Goh, C. & Agius, M. (2020) The stress-vulnerability model how does stress impact on mental illness at the level of the brain and what are the consequences? *Psychiatria Danubina* 22(2), 198–202.

Hammersley, P., Read, J. & Dillon, J. (2008) Childhood trauma and psychosis: The genie is out of the bottle. *Journal of Psychological Trauma* 6(2–3), 7–20. http://dx.doi.org/10.1300/J513v06n02_02

Health Service Executive (2023) *Mental Health Engagement and Recovery Office Strategic Plan 2023-2026: Engaged in Recovery* (Internet). Available at: www.hse.ie/eng/services/list/4/mental-health-services/mental-health-engagement-and-recovery/resources-information-and-publications/a-national-framework-for-recovery-in-mental-health.pdf (accessed 09 September 2024).

Health Service Executive (2024) *A National Framework for Recovery in Mental Health: 2024-2028* (Internet). Available at: www.hse.ie/eng/services/list/4/mental-health- services/mental-health-engagement-and-recovery/resources-information-and-publications/a-national-framework-for-recovery-in-mental-health.pdf (accessed 09 September 2024).

Herman, J.L. (2001) *Trauma and Recovery: From Domestic Abuse to Political Terror.* Pandora, London.

Hickney, W. (2022) *The Early Peer Support Movement* (Internet). Available at: https://cmwn.org/the-history-of-peer-support/the-early-peer-support-movement/#:~:text=With out%20the%20efforts%20of%20early,very%20first%20peer %2Drun%20organizations (accessed 09 September 2024).

Huda, A.S. (2019) *The Medical Model in Mental Health: An Explanation and Evaluation.* Oxford University Press, Oxford.

Hunt, E. & Byrne, M. (2019) *Peer Support Workers in Mental Health Services: A Report on the Impact of Peer Support Workers in Mental Health Services* (Internet). Available at: www.lenus.ie/bitstream/handle/10147/635104/peer-support-workers-in-mental-health-services.pdf?sequence=1&isAllowed=y (accessed 22 September 2024).

Kalachanis, K. & Michailidis, I.E. (2015) The Hippocratic view on humors and human temperament. *European Journal of Social Behaviour* 2(2), 1–5.

Kalachanis, K. & Tsagkaris, C. (2020) The Hippocratic account of mental health: Humors and human temperament. *Mental Health: Global Challenges Journal* 3(1), 33–37. https://doi.org/10.32437/mhgcj.v3i1.83

Karter, J. (2024) *Global Mental Health Leaders Shift Away from Biomedical Model Towards Rights-Based Approaches* (Internet). Available at: www.madinamerica.com/2024/06/glo bal-mental-health-leaders-shift-away-from-biomedical-model-towards-rights-based-app roaches/ (accessed 22 September 2024).

Kelly, B. (2019) *Hearing Voices: The History of Psychiatry in Ireland.* Irish Academic Press, Kildare.

Kelly, B. (2022a) *In Search of Madness: A Psychiatrist's Travels through the History of Mental Illness.* Gill Books, Ireland.

Kelly, B. (2022b) *Building A Better Mental Health Service* (Internet). Available at: www.med icalindependent.ie/comment/opinion/building-a-better-mental-health-service/ (accessed 25 August 2024).

Kelly, T. (2020) *Bealach Nua – Supporting Families of People with Mental Health Difficulties* (Internet). Available at: www.con-telegraph.ie/2020/12/08/bealach-nua-supporting-famil ies-of-people-with-mental-health-difficulties/ (accessed 22 September 2024).

Kinser, P.A. & Lyon, D.E. (2014) A conceptual framework of stress vulnerability, depression and health outcomes in women: Potential uses in research on complementary therapies for depression. *Brain and Behavior* 4(5), 665–674. https://doi.org/10.1002/brb3.249

Lagay, F. (2002) The legacy of humoral medicine. *AMA Journal of Ethics* 4(7), 206–208. https://doi.org/10.1001/virtualmentor.2002.4.7.mhst1-0207.

Lempesis, I.G., Georgakopoulou, V.K., Chrousos, G.P. & Spandidos, D.A. (2024) Bridging ancient wisdom and contemporary medicine science: Contemplating on Hippocrates theory of humours. *World Academy of Sciences Journal* 6(2), 18. https://doi.org/10.3892/ wasj.2024.233

Mahon, D. (2022) *Trauma-Responsive Organisations: The Trauma Ecology Model.* Emerald Publishing Limited, Bingley.

Moore, J. (2020) *John Read and Irving Kirsch – Electroconvulsive Therapy (ECT) Does the Evidence from Clinical Trials Justify its Continued Use?* (Internet) Available at: www. madinamerica.com/2020/06/john-read-irving-kirsch-electroconvulsive-therapy-ect-evide nce-clinical-trials-justify-continued-use/ (accessed 08 September 2024).

Norton, M.J. (2019) Implementing co-production in traditional statutory mental health ser- vices. *Mental Health Practice.* https://doi.org/10.7748/mhp.2019.e1304

Norton, M.J. (2021) Co-production within child and adolescent mental health: A system- atic review. *International Journal of Environmental Research and Public Health* 18(22), 11897. https://doi.org/10.3390/ijerph182211897

Norton, M.J. (2022) *Co-Production in Mental Health: Implementing Policy into Practice.* Routledge, Abingdon.

Norton, M.J. (2023a) 'A National Framework for Mental Health Engagement and Recovery': A Co-designed Measurement Tool (MSc Dissertation). Royal College of Surgeons in Ireland, Dublin, Ireland.

Norton, M.J. (2023b) Mental health peer-led cafés – A complimentary approach to trad- itional crisis care: A protocol for a systematic scoping reivew. *Psychiatry International* 4, 370–379. https://doi.org/10.3390/psychiatryint4040033

Norton, M.J. (2024) Peer work in mental health services. In *Peer Support Work: Practice, Training and Implementation* (Mahon, D. ed.) Emerald Publishing Limited, Leeds, pp. 9–23.

Norton, M.J. & Cullen, O.J. (2024) Contextual and personal introduction to the text. In *Different Diagnoses, Similar Experiences: Narratives of Mental Health, Addiction Recovery and Dual Diagnosis* (Norton, M.J. & Cullen, O.J. eds.), Emerald Publishing Limited, Leeds, pp. 3–18.

Norton, M.J., Griffin, M., Collins, M., Clark, M. & Browne, E. (2023) Using autoethnography to reflect on peer support supervision in an Irish context. *The Journal of Practice Teaching and Learning* 21(1-2). https://doi.org/10.1921/jpts.v21i2.2079

Oireachtas (2024) *Mental Health Bill 2024* (Internet). Available at: https://data.oireachtas.ie/ie/oireachtas/bill/2024/66/eng/initiated/b6624d.pdf (accessed 25 August 2024).

Patel, V., Saxena, S., Lund, C., Kohrt, B., Kieling, C., Sunkel, C., Kola, L., Chang, O., Charlson, F., O'Neill, K. & Herrman, H. (2023) Transforming mental health systems globally: Principles and policy recommendations. *The Lancet* 402(10402), 656–666. https://doi.org/10.1016/S0140-6736(23)00918-2

Read, J. (2013) Childhood adversity and psychosis: From heresy to certainty. In *Models of Madness: Psychological, Social and biological Approaches to Psychosis* (Read, J. & Dillon, J. eds.) Routledge, East Sussex, pp. 249–275.

Read, J. & Bentall, R. (2010) The effectiveness of electroconvulsive therapy: A literature review. *Social Psychiatry and Psychiatric Epidemiology* 19(4), 333–347. https://doi.org/10.1017/s1121189x00000671

Read, J. & Dillon, J. (2013) *Models of Madness: Psychological, Social and Biological Approaches to Psychosis* (2nd edn), Routledge, East Sussex.

Read, J., Kirsch, I. & McGrath, L. (2020) Electroconvulsive therapy for depression: A review of the quality of ECT versus sham ECT trials and meta-analyses. *Ethical Human Psychology and Psychiatry* 21(2), EHPP-D-19-00014. https://doi.org/10.1891/EHPP-D-19- 00014

Richter, D. & Dixon, J. (2023) Models of mental health problems: A quasi-systematic review of theoretical approaches. *Journal of Mental Health* 32(2), 394–406. https://doi.org/10.1080/09638237.2021.2022638

Salicru, S. (2020) Retiring categorical systems and the biomedical model of mental illness: The why and the how – A clinician's perspective. *Psychology* 11(8), 1215–1235. https://doi.org/10.4236/psych.2020.118081

SAMHSA's Trauma and Justice Strategic Initiative (2014) *SAMHSA's Concept of Trauma and Guidance for a Trauma-Informed Approach* (Internet). Available at: https://library.samhsa.gov/sites/default/files/sma14-4884.pdf (accessed 22 September 2024).

Shalaby, R.A.H. & Agyapong, V.I.O. (2020) Peer support in mental health: Literature review. *JMIR Mental Health* 7(6), e15572. https://doi.org/10.2196/15572.

Taylor, J. & Shrive, J. (2024) *Indicative Trauma Impact Manual: A Non-Diagnostic, Trauma-Informed Guide to Emotion, Thought and Behaviour*. VictinFocus Ltd, United Kingdom.

The Stationary Office (1984) *The Psychiatric Services – Planning for the Future: Report of a Study Group on the Development of the Psychiatric Services* (Internet) Available at: www.lenus.ie/handle/10147/45556 (accessed 08 September 2024).

Thompson, J.W. (1994) Trends in the development of psychiatric services, 1844–1994. *Hospital and Community Psychiartry* 45(10), 987–992.

Van Der Kolk, B. (2015) *The Body Keeps the Score: Mind, Brain and Body in the Transformation of Trauma*. Penguin Books, United States of America.

Watson, J. (2017) *Time to 'Drop the Disorder'* (Internet). Available at: www.madinamerica.com/2017/01/time-drop-disorder/ (accessed 08 September 2024).

Yapijakis, C. (2009) Hippocrates of Kos, the father of clinical medicine and Asclepiades of Bithynia, the father of molecular medicine. *In Vivo* 23, 507–514.

Young, C. (2024) *Talking Trauma: Trying to be Heard over Toxic Trauma Rhetoric* (Internet). Available at: www.centreformentalhealth.org.uk/talking-trauma-trying-to-be-heard-over-toxic-trauma-rhetoric/ (available 29 September 2024).

Zunes, S. & Laird, J. (2010) *The US Civil Rights Movement (1942–1968)* (Internet). Available at: www.nonviolent-conflict.org/us-civil-rights-movement-1942-1968/ (accessed 08 September 2024).

Chapter 3

Definitions of Peer Support Work

3.1 Introduction

In the previous two chapters, the focus centred on contextualising peer support work within both mental health service provision and an Irish context. These previous chapters not only examined the current makeup of the mental health services both in Ireland and abroad but additionally, for the purposes of orientation, drew our attention to what had occurred in the past. All these allowed us to note that both recovery and the modern peer support movement developed as a result of activism both within and external to the mental health space.

This chapter aims to enhance what has been discovered previously by examining the elements needed to construct a definition for peer support work specifically aimed for use within mental health service provision. The need for such discussions has increased dramatically as the peer movement has progressively gained traction as a model that, at its core, allows services to meet the needs of the communities they serve (Quality Matters, 2023). However, as noted already in the literature base, peer support work is difficult to conceptually pin down due to the variety of definitions that already exist both externally and internally for mental health service provision (Shalaby and Agyapong, 2020) but also because of its complex and unsteady foundations which are particularly founded within mental health discourse (Davidson et al., 2012; von Peter et al., 2024).

This chapter is structured as follows: Section 3.2 examines various understandings of peer support work already noted in the literature. In essence, this section extracts key aspects that are vital to construct a new definition. This construction then takes place in Section 3.3. Finally, Section 3.4 concludes this chapter by summarising the learnings that are extrapolated from this chapter and also providing a brief glimpse into what will follow in the forthcoming chapters of this book.

3.2 Defining Peer Support Work

As noted by Mahon (2024), peers are not a homogenous group; rather, they use common processes to provide support and engagement to individuals with a variety

DOI: 10.4324/9781032717050-5

of social and health care–associated needs. Indeed, in recent times, peer support work has increasingly been integrated into mental health services to help people with lived experiences of mental health recover from these challenges (Poremski et al., 2022). However, at the time of writing in 2024, there is a lack of definitional clarity for peer support work in mental health service provision (Shalaby and Agyapong, 2020; Dayan, 2022; Norton, 2024a). There are a number of reasons for this: varied modalities of peer support work within mental health discourse currently, as described in Table 3.1 (Stefancic et al., 2021; Simmons et al., 2023; Robertson et al., 2024); its historical underpinnings which are mainly situated within Western cultures, where most of the research pertaining to peer support as a concept also lies (Gillard et al., 2013; Kuek et al., 2021); the unhelpful interchange-ability of peer support work as a term with other similar concepts like *'consumer services'*, *'peer specialists'* and *'peer workers'* (Penney, 2018).

As peer support represents a wide range of activities, it is important for this par-ticular text to have a focus even at this basic level. This focus will be on formalised or intentional peer support work activity delivered by those with lived experience who are paid and trained to use this experience to help others recover. Simpson et al. (2017) note that this is a relatively new development in mental health dis-course. Despite its novelty in service provision, it already has piqued the interest of scholars across the world, with one recent paper describing the intervention as low-threshold, benefiting individual service users by enhancing empowerment and personal recovery-related outcomes (Nixdorf et al., 2024). Another work by Wyder et al. (2020) has also noted how formalised peer workers are an ever-expanding component of the mental health workforce. However, before one can explore for-malised/intentional peer support work further, an appropriate definition for this text must be constructed based on key components described in the already-published literature regarding peer support work.

3.2.1 Key Components in the Published Definitions on Formalised Peer Support Work in Mental Health

The concept of peer support work through a formalised lens cannot or should not be defined through one singular sentence or approach (Ahluwalia, 2018). This chapter recognises that formalised peer support work is characterised in many dif-ferent ways depending on the context by which it is being used. As a result it also acknowledges that the literature has yet to construct a universal definition that can be used across the formalised peer support sector. In an attempt to do so, an exam-ination of the peer support work literature was conducted, examining specifically the various components that make up a definition. What was revealed was that, while definitions varied, they all had several components that played a central role in the construction of the definition (see Table 3.2). Each component is described in the following sections.

Firstly, peer support is described as both a **one-directional** (Davidson et al. 2006; Faulkner and Basset, 2010) and **reciprocal process** (Mead et al., 2001; Barlow

Table 3.1 Different Modalities of Peer Support Work in Mental Health

Model	Description	Delivery Methods	Specific Model Benefits
One-on-one (individual)	Peer support between two people. Most likely involving a professional third party to link the two people together	Face to face, via phone, online	Tailored for the individual
Group peer-to-peer support	Groups share a lived experience. May be structured and organised, however, no formal facilitator. Can be independent or tied to a larger network	Face to face, online	Tailored to the shared lived experience. Can be informal and include social activities
Peer-led groups	Peer leaders share their lived experience to support and educate others similar to themselves. Can be workshops or structured group peer support often tied to a larger network	Face to face, online	Tailored to the shared lived experience. May have educational aspects
Groups co-facilitated by peer and traditionally qualified experts (e.g. clinicians)	Often involves professional health services, where a group of people with a shared lived experience are supported by both an expert and peer. Can be structured and formal	Face to face, online	Tailored to both group and individual. May have educational and treatment aspects
Online peer support	Can be one-on-one or group format. May have professional involvement through moderators. Mostly peer-to-peer support through forums	Online	Can be anonymous

Source: Adapted from Simmons et al. (2023).

Table 3.2 Key Components for Defining Formalised Peer Support Work

No.	Key Components	Explanation
1.	One-directional or reciprocal	A one-way process.
		A reciprocal process where both the service user and Peer Support Worker support each other through their recovery processes.
2.	Reflective	Allowing an individual peer to reflect on their lived experiences.
3.	Formalised	In a formalised, paid role within the mental health services which aligns them to uphold the vision, mission and subsequent values of the organisation.
4.	Trained role	Individual peers are trained to a certain standard – differs per country – to offer support through the sharing of lived experience.
5.	Lived experience	Experiences that are transformed into a knowledge set that can then be used to support other in their own recovery.
6.	Provide social and emotional support	Supports a person with regard to their mental health and re-integration back as a meaningful and contributing member of society.
7.	One-to-one or group-based support	Can occur on either a one-to-one or through a peer support group capacity.
8.	Mutual agreement	With those who self-identify as having or had a mental health challenge to those with similar challenges.
9.	Diagnosis	Of what is helpful. Does not have to be the same as those they support.
10.	Understand another person's situation empathetically	To examine ones' life circumstances in an empathetic manner where support and care are seen as key.
12.	Provide support to a person caring for someone	To support the supporter in their caring role.
13.	Assist in their recovery	So that they can live a life that is meaningful and purposeful to them, whatever that looks like for them.

et al., 2010; Department of Health, 2020). In reciprocal process, two groups of individuals/communities rely on each other for a mutual service (Beltran et al., 2023). This becomes one-directional due to the professionalisation of the peer role, which will be discussed in Chapter 8. Next, and perhaps surprisingly, only one paper (Bouchard et al., 2010) suggested that peer support work is **a reflective process** that allows individuals to look back on their experiences, and on their interactions, they can utilise both to enhance future encounters within their practice. The lack of authors stating the reflective nature of the role is surprising, considering that other professionals within mental health discourse, like nursing, have reflective practice as a core competency of their practice and additionally as an essential aspect of their registration in a country of interest by a professional body (Nursing and Midwifery Board of Ireland, 2015; Tolosa-Merlos et al., 2023).

Faulkner and Basset (2010), Chang et al. (2016) and Kuek et al. (2021) all suggest that peer support work in this context should be **formalised**. Formalisation refers to the professionalisation of the role both through formal, accredited **training** and through the creation of a set of principles, standards, governance structures and a process for accreditation and maintaining up-to-date professional practice – all of which are identified mechanisms of professionalism as stipulated by Wilensky's (1964) seminal work on professionalisation. Perhaps the largest cited aspect of a peer support work definition through a formalised lens is the presence of **lived experience** of mental health difficulties (Davidson et al., 2006; Coniglio et al., 2012; Austin et al., 2014; Chang et al., 2016; Myrick and del Vecchio, 2016; Daniels et al., 2017; Hunt and Byrne, 2019; Leemeijer and Noordegraaf, 2020; Kuek et al., 2021; World Health Organisation, 2021; Fortuna et al., 2022; Norton et al., 2023; Walde et al., 2023) or lived experience of caring for someone with mental health challenges (Norton et al., 2023). The reason for the aspect is lived experience – transformed into a knowledge set (experiential knowledge) that is used by the peer to create connections, introduce informality and enable the individual service user/family member to be provided with the **social and emotional supports** necessary for them to once again dream about the future and reflect on what recovery looks like for them (Repper et al., 2013; Norton, 2022, 2023; Fortuna et al., 2022; Norton, 2024b).

Such social and emotional supports can be delivered through a variety of mechanisms, including on a **one-to-one** level or through a **group-based** peer support programme with formalised peers (Davidson et al., 2006; Barlow et al., 2010; Faulkner and Basset, 2010; World Health Organisation, 2021). In addition, these supports are given through a **mutual agreement** that (1) both individuals self-identify as having/had a mental health or other similar challenges (Mead et al., 2001; Soloman, 2004; Barlow et al., 2010; Repper et al., 2013; Walker and Bryant, 2013; Blash et al., 2015; Puschner et al., 2019; Department of Health, 2020; World Health Organisation, 2021; Fortuna et al., 2022) and (2) the programme of work that would be most helpful to the person receiving support (Mead et al., 2001; Department of Health, 2020). Such mutual mental health challenges as highlighted by Mead et al. (2001), Soloman (2004), Barlow et al. (2010), Repper et al. (2013),

Walker and Bryant (2013), Blash et al. (2015), Puschner et al. (2019), Department of Health (2020), World Health Organisation (2021) and Fortuna et al. (2022) do not mean that the peer supporters have to have the same **diagnosis** as those they are supporting (Wall et al., 2022). Instead, what is more important is that the peer can reach a level of **understanding of a person's situation that allows them to approach the situation and the service user/family member empathetically** (Department of Health, 2020). All of these serve one of two purposes: (1) to **assist a service user in their individualised recovery journey** (Austin et al., 2014; Daniels et al., 2017; Hunt and Byrne, 2019; Leemeijer and Noordegraaf, 2020; Fortuna et al., 2022; Wadle et al., 2023) or (2) to **provide support to a person caring for a loved one with mental health difficulties** (Norton et al., 2023).

3.3 A Definition of Peer Support Work to Be Used in This Text

As identified above, peer support work, when observed through a formalised lens, has several components that can be used to creatively construct a new, novel definition for the concept. From which the following definition was constructed, suggesting that peer support work in mental health is defined as follows:

A formalised process that can be either one-directional or reciprocal which is carried out through trained, reflective practitioners who therapeutically utilises their own lived experiences of mental health challenges to provide social and emotional support – either through one-on-one or group based – through a mutual agreement of self-expression as a person with mental health challenges, regardless of diagnosis, where such individuals can understand another person's situation empathetically to either provide support to those caring for another with mental health difficulties or to assist the service user themselves in attaining recovery, whatever that may look like for them.

3.4 Concluding Remarks

This chapter aimed to develop a new definition for peer support work which could then be used to shape the remaining chapters. This construction was made possible by a thorough examination of existing definitions within the mental health literature to identify key components that were most prominent and necessary for inclusion in any new definition of peer support work. From which, this new definition reflects the current necessary components identified in the literature as to peer support work in mental health discourse. Only time will tell if this definition will remain valid and useful to the academic community – which may be difficult to ascertain given the increasing interest in this field of study. The next chapter will expand on some of these key components highlighted above as well as discuss various principles and roles associated with formalised peer support work in mental health service provision.

References

Ahluwalia, A. (2018) *Peer Support in Practice: A Research Report with Recommendations for Practice* (Internet). Available at: www.drilluk.org.uk/wp- content/uploads/2018/02/Peer-Support-in-Practice-Final-Inclusion-Barnet-2018.pdf (Accessed 20 October 2024).

Austin, E., Ramakrishnan, A. & Hopper, K. (2014) Embodying recovery: A qualitative study of peer work in a consumer-run service setting. *Community Mental Health Journal* 50(8), 879–885. https://doi.org/10.1007/s10597-014-9693-z

Barlow, C.A., Schiff, J.W., Chugh, U., Rawlinson, D., Hides, E. & Leith, J. (2010) An evaluation of a suicide bereavement peer support program. *Death Studies* 34(10), 915–930. https://doi.org/10.1080/07481181003761435

Beltran, D.G., Ayers, J.D., Munoz, A., Cronk, L. & Aktipis, A. (2023) What is reciprocity? A review and expert-based classification of cooperative transfers. *Evolution and Human Behavior*. https://doi.org/10.1016/j.evolhumbehav.2023.05.003

Blash, L., Chan, K. & Chapman, S. (2015) *The Peer Provider Workforce in Behavioural Health: A Landscape Analysis* (Internet). Available at: https://healthworkforce.ucsf.edu/sites/healthworkforce.ucsf.edu/files/Report-Peer_Provider_Workforce_in_Behavioral_Health-A_Landscape_Analysis.pdf (Accessed 20th October 2024).

Bouchard, L., Montreuil, M. & Gros, C. (2010) Peer support among inpatients in an adult mental health setting. *Issues in Mental Health Nursing* 31, 589–598. https://doi.org/10.3109/01612841003793049

Chang, B-H., Mueller, L., Resnick, S.G., Osatuke, K. & Eisen, S.V. (2016) Job satisfaction of department of veteran affairs peer mental health providers. *Psychiatric Rehabilitation Journal* 39(1), 47–54. https://doi.org/10.1037/prj0000162

Coniglio, F.D., Hancock, N. & Ellis, L.A. (2012) Peer support within clubhouse: A grounded theory study. *Community Mental Health Journal* 48, 153–160. https://doi.org/10.1007/s10597- 010-9358-5

Daniels, A.S., Bergeson, S. & Myrick, K.J. (2017) Defining peer roles and status among community health workers and peer support specialists in integrated systems of care. *Psychiatric Services* 68(12), 1296–1298. https://doi.org/10.1176/appi.ps.201600378

Davidson, L., Bellamy, C., Guy, K. & Miller, R. (2012) Peer support among persons with severe mental illnesses: A review of evidence and experience. *World Psychiatry* 11(2), 123–128. https://doi.org/10.1016/j.wpsyc.2012.05.009

Davidson, L., Chinman, M., Sells, D. & Rowe, M. (2006) Peer support among adults with serious mental illness: A report from the field. *Schizophrenia Bulletin* 32, 443–450. https://doi.org/10.1093/schbul/sbj043

Dayan, E. (2022) *Peer Support Research: Is It Time Yet?* (Internet) Available at: www.madinamerica.com/2022/05/peer-support-research/ (Accessed 17 October 2024).

Department of Health (2020) *Sharing the Vision: A Mental Health Policy for Everyone* (Internet). Available at: https://assets.gov.ie/static/documents/sharing-the-vision-a-mental-health-policy-for-everyone.pdf (Accessed 19 October 2024).

Faulkner, A. & Basset T. (2010) *A Helping Hand: Consultations with Service Users about Peer Support* (Internet). Available at: www.together-uk.org/wp-content/uploads/2023/08/A-helping-hand-consultation-with-service-users-about-peer- support.pdf (Accessed 20 October 2024).

Fortuna, K.L., Solomon, P. & Rivera, J. (2022) An update of peer support/peer provided services underlying processes, benefits, and critical ingredients. *Psychiatric Quarterly* 93(2), 571–586. https://doi.org/10.1007/s11126-022-09971-w

Gillard, S.G., Edwards, C., Gibson, S.L., Owen, K. & Wright, C. (2013) Introducing peer worker roles into UK mental health service teams: A qualitative analysis of the organisational benefits and challenges. *BMC Health Services Research* 13, 188. https://doi.org/10.1186/1472-6963-13-188

Hunt, E. & Byrne, M. (2019) *Peer Support Workers in Mental Health Services: A Report on the Impact of Peer Support Workers in Mental Health Services* (Internet). Available at: www.lenus.ie/bitstream/handle/10147/635104/peer-support-workers-in-mental-health-services.pdf?sequence=1&isAllowed=y (Accessed 19 October 2024).

Kuek, J.H.L., Chua, H.C. & Poremski, D. (2021) Barriers and facilitators of peer support work in a large psychiatric hospital: A thematic analysis. *General Psychiatry* 34(3), e100521. https://doi.org/10.1136/gpsych-2021-100521

Leemeijer, A. & Noordegraaf, M. (2020) Health professionals and peer support workers in mental health settings. In *Support Workers and the Health Professions in International Perspective: The Invisible Providers of Health Care* (Saks, M. ed.). Policy Press, Bristol, pp. 143–160.

Mahon, D. (2024) Peer support work: A brief introduction. In *Peer Support Work: Practice, Training and Implementation* (Mahon, D. ed.). Emerald Publishing Limited, Leeds, pp. 3–8.

Mead, S., Hilton, D. & Curtis, L. (2001) Peer support: A theoretical perspective. *Psychiatric Rehabilitation Journal* 25(2), 134–141. https://doi.org/10.1037/h0095032

Myrick, K. & del Vecchio, P. (2016) Peer support services in the behavioural healthcare workforce: State of the field. *Psychiatric Rehabilitation Journal* 39(3), 197–203. http://dx.doi.org/10.1037/prj0000188

Nixdorf, R., Kotera, Y., Baillie, D., Epstein, P.G., Hall, C., Hiltensperger, R., Korde, P., Moran, G., Mpango, R., Nakku, J., Puschner, B., Ramesh, M., Repper, J., Shamba, D., Slade, M., Kalha, J. & Mahlke, C. (2024) Development of the UPSIDES global mental health training programme for peer support workers: Perspectives from stakeholders in low, middle and high-income countries. *PLOS ONE* 19(2), e0298315. https://doi.org/10.1371/journal.pone.0298315

Norton, M.J. (2022) More than just a health care assistant: Peer support working within rehabilitation and recovery mental health services. *Irish Journal of Psychological Medicine*. https://doi.org/10.1017/ipm.2022.32

Norton, M.J. (2023) Peer support working: A question of ontology and epistemology? *International Journal of Mental Health Systems* 17, 1. https://doi.org/10.1186/s13033-023-00570-1

Norton, M.J. (2024a) Peer work in mental health services. In *Peer Support Work: Practice, Training and Implementation* (Mahon, D. ed.). Emerald Publishing Limited, Leeds, pp. 9–23.

Norton, M.J. (2024b) Using learned tools for experiential gain: The application of experiential knowledge to traditional service processes. *Irish Journal of Psychological Medicine*. https://doi.org/10.1017/ipm.2024.4

Norton, M.J., Clabby, P., Coyle, B., Cruickshank, J., Davidson, G., Greer, K., Kilcommins, M., McCartan, C., McGuire, E., McGilloway, S., Mulholland, C., O'Connell-Gannon, M., Pepper, D., Shannon, C., Swords, C., Walsh, J. & Webb, P. (2023) *Peer Support Work: An International Scoping Review* (Internet). Available at: https://pureadmin.qub.ac.uk/ws/portalfiles/portal/543700214/Peer_Support_Work_Scoping_Review_Main_report.pdf (Accessed 19 October 2024).

Nursing and Midwifery Board of Ireland (2015) *Scope of Nursing and Midwifery Practice Framework* (Internet). Available at: www.nmbi.ie/nmbi/media/NMBI/Publications/Scope-of-Nursing-Midwifery-Practice-Framework.pdf?ext=.pdf (Accessed 20 October 2024).

Penney, D. (2018) *Who Gets to Define "Peer Support?"* (Internet). Available at: www.madin america.com/2018/02/who-gets-to-define-peer-support/ (Accessed 17 October 2024).

Poremski, D., Kuek, J.H.L., Yuan, Q., Li, Z., Yaw, K.L., Eu, P.W. & Chua, H.C. (2022) The impact of peer support work on the mental health of peer support specialists. *International Journal of Mental Health Systems* 16, 51. https://doi.org/10.1186/s13033-022-00561-8

Puschner, B., Repper, J., Mahlke, C., Nixdorf, R., Basangwa, D., Nakku, J., Ryan, G., Baillie, D., Shamba, D., Ramesh, M., Moran, G., Lachmann, M., Kalha, J., Pathare, S., Muller- Stierlin, A. & Slade, M. (2019) Using peer support in developing empowering mental health services (UPSIDES): Background, rationale and methodology. *Annals of Global Health* 85(1), 53. https://doi.org/10.5334/aogh.2435

Quality Matters (2023) *Doing Peer Work: An Introductory Guide to Co-Designing Peer Work Roles or Programmes in your Service* (Internet). Available at: www.drugsandalco hol.ie/38913/1/Doing_peer_work_guide_2023.pdf (Accessed 16 October 2024).

Repper, J., Aldridge, B., Gilfoyle, S., Gillard, S., Perkins, R. & Rennison, J. (2013) *Peer Support Workers: Theory and Practice* (Internet). Available at: https://static1.squaresp ace.com/static/65e873c27971d37984653be0/t/668ce21ba54f933596890e57/172050 8956537/5ImROC-Peer-Support-Workers-Theory-and-Practice.pdf (Accessed 20 October 2024).

Robertson, S., Leigh-Phippard, H., Robertson, D., Thomson, A., Casey, J. & Walsh, L.J. (2024) What supports the emotional well-being of peer workers in an NHS mental health service? *Mental Health and Social Inclusion.* https://doi.org/10.1108/MHSI-02-2024-0023

Shalaby, R.A.H. & Agyapong, V.I.O. (2020) Peer support in mental health – A general review of the literature. *JMIR Mental Health* 7(6), e15572. https://doi.org/10.2196/15572

Simmons, M.B., Cartner, S., MacDonald, R., Whitson, S., Bailey, A. & Brown, E. (2023) The effectiveness of peer support from a person with lived experience of mental health challenges for young people with anxiety and depression: A systematic review. *BMC Psychiatry* 13, 194. https://doi.org/10.1186/s12888-023-04578-2

Simpson, A., Oster, C. & Muir-Cochrane, E. (2017) Liminality in the occupational iden-tity of mental health peer support workers: A qualitative study. *International Journal of Mental Health Nursing* 27(2), 662–671. https://doi.org/10.1111/inm.12351

Solomon, P. (2004) Peer support/peer guided services: Underlying processes, benefits and critical ingredients. *Psychiatric Rehabilitation Journal* 27, 392–401. https://doi.org/10.2975/27.2004.392.401

Stefancic, A., Bochicchio, L. & Tuda, D. (2021) Peer support in mental health. In *Peer Support in Medicine: A Quick Guide* (Avery, J.D. ed.). Springer Nature, Switzerland, pp. 31–48.

Tolosa-Merlos, D., Moreno-Poyato, A.R., Gonzalez-Palau, F., Perez-Toribio, A., Casanova-Garrigos, G., Delgado-Hito, P. & MiRTCIME.CAT Working Group (2023) Exploring the therapeutic relationship through the reflective practice of nurses in acute mental health units: A qualitative Study. *Journal of Clinical Nursing* 32(1–2), 253–263. https://doi.org/10.1111/jocn.16223

von Peter, S., Lraemwe, U.M., Cubellis, L., Fehler, G., Ruiz-Perez, G., Schmidt, D., Ziegenhagen, J., Kuesel, M., Ackers, S., Mahlke, C., Nugent, L. & Heuer, I. (2024) Implementing peer support work in mental health carer in Germany: The methodological framework of the collaborative, participatory, mixed-methods study (ImpPeer-Psy5). *Health Expectations* 27(1), e13938. https://doi.org/10.1111/hex.13938

Wadle, P., Hadala, J., Peipe, V. & Vollm, B.A. (2023) Implementation of a peer support worker in a forensic psychiatric hospital in Germany – Views of patients. *Frontiers in Psychiatry* 14, 1061106. https://doi.org/10.3389/fpsyt.2023.1061106

Walker, G. & Bryant, W. (2013) Peer support in adult mental health services: A metasynthesis of qualitative findings. *Psychiatric Rehabilitation Journal* 36(1), 28–34. https://doi.org/10.1037/h0094744

Wall, A., Lovheden, T., Landgren, K. & Stjernsward, S. (2022) Experience and challenges in the role as peer support workers in a Swedish mental health context – An interview study. *Issues in Mental Health Nursing* 43(4), 344–355. https://doi.org/10.1080/01612840.2021.1978596

Wilensky, H.L. (1964) The professionalization of everyone? *The American Journal of Sociology* 70(2), 137–158.

World Health Organisation (2021) *Peer Support Mental Health Services: Promoting Person- Centred and Rights-Based Approaches* (Internet). Available at: https://iris.who.int/bitstream/handle/10665/341643/9789240025783- eng.pdf?sequence=1 (Accessed 19 October 2024).

Wyder, M., Roennfeldt, H., Parker, S., Vilic, G., McCann, K., Ehrlich, C. & Dark, F.L. (2020) Diary of a mental health peer worker: Findings from a diary study into the role of peer work in a clinical mental health setting. *Frontiers of Psychiatry* 11, 587656. https://doi.org/10.3389/fpsyt.2020.587656

Chapter 4

Principles and Roles of Peer Support Work

Case Study Contributors:

Sandra O'Sullivan, William Gallini-Poole, and Olga Zilberberg

4.1 Introduction

According to Naughton et al. (2015) and Gray and Sisto (2024), the peer's role is to utilise their inherent shared lived experiences to support an individual in their recovery journey. However, the mechanism by which this experience is shared is still a matter of some debate (Norton, 2022; Archard et al., 2023). A similar debate is evident for many of the other roles associated with peer support work, which has led to a well-documented and long-standing position that peer support work has been and is currently still debated. That is the lack of role clarity (Kemp and Henderson, 2012; Adams et al., 2023; Glynn, 2023; Reeves et al., 2024). This long-standing issue needs to be addressed as Abraham and colleagues found that there is a statistically significant causal link between the lack of role clarity experienced by multiple stakeholders towards peer roles and the emotional exhaustion that is experienced by these same peers, which leads to burnout. All of this, in turn, inhibits the peer's integration into multi-disciplinary teams, leading to indefinite leaves of absence from work (Jacobson et al., 2012). As such, organisations need to address this lack of role clarity along with issues pertaining to supervision, professional development and perceived lack of value to better support peer support work within services (Stefancic et al., 2021).

This chapter aims to address this lack of clarity regarding the roles and functions of Peer Support Workers in mental health through a number of lenses. The chapter begins in Section 4.2 by exploring various principles of peer support work. Principles in this context relate to various values a peer is expected to hold as part of their work. This is an important element as the roles of the peer are directly linked with the peer's value system/principles that underpin their work (Gillard et al., 2017). This is then followed by Section 4.3 which explores various roles of the peer, in so doing, explaining why some roles may be similar to other professionals within the mental health field but coming from a different position and lens. Both Sections 4.2 and 4.3 are supported by case studies from external contributors who practise, in one degree or another, peer work in mental health service provision. The chapter concludes with Section 4.4 where a summary is presented along with links to the following chapter of this book.

DOI: 10.4324/9781032717050-6

4.2 Principles of Peer Support Work

A principle is defined as a type of belief, rule or idea that guides persons and their practices (Vocabulary.com, 2024). Within the context of peer support work, there are a number of core principles that govern how peer professionals like Peer Support Workers carry out their roles and maintain authenticity in their actions (Repper et al., 2013). The principles highlighted below are non-exhaustive; rather they represent the core principles of peer support work highlighted within the literature, which is necessary for peer support work to actually make a difference in a person's life. These principles are described below through narrative inquiry and the use of case studies.

4.2.1 Mutuality

Mutuality is a concept that occurs through an interactional accomplishment of enactment that sits on a continuum between tight and loose emotional management which occurs over different objects, strategies and with varying levels of intensity (Kirkegaard and Andersen, 2022). Simply put, it is about people with similar life experiences coming together, sharing strategies and techniques and ultimately supporting each other authentically through each other's respective mental health challenges (Faulkner et al., 2013). The simplicity of mutuality has become one of the key principles of peer support work (Paulson et al., 1999), and indeed, it can be said that the entire peer relationship is built upon the principle of mutuality itself (Hunt and Byrne, 2019). In essence what ultimately creates mutuality is the sharing of each other's lived experiences of mental health challenges and subsequent recovery (Cabral et al., 2014; Rosenberg and Argentzell, 2018). This sharing of lived experiences also has a therapeutic purpose as it provides the service user with a sense of validation and comfort in recognising that they are not suffering alone (Barr et al., 2020). As noted earlier, mutuality occurs through the sharing of narratives. In our first case study, Sandra, a newly qualified peer from Ireland, describes how she practises mutuality in her own peer support practice in her own words.

Case Study 1   Practising Mutuality in Peer Support

Sandra O'Sullivan

I am a Peer Support Worker who studied in Dublin City University studying peer support during the period 2022–2023 and worked on placement as a Peer Support Worker in Limerick Mental Health Association during this time. I am discussing practising mutuality as a peer and how I achieved this as part of my work experience. In achieving this I utilised my lived experience as a person who had previously endured mental health difficulties and experienced recovery in my support of peers.

I created a space for dialogue between myself and the peer I was supporting to enable mutual experiences and perspectives to be explored. This dialogue has been created to enable this mutual experience and different perspectives to be shared. I share my story with peers and build mutuality. To foster the growth of mutuality, I will demonstrate active listening and use my own interpersonal skills such as empathy, verbal communication and non-verbal communication to foster hope, identity and empowerment. I will also use my personal narrative/lived experience to strategically share my story with peers to build mutuality.

In creating mutuality between myself and my peers, I used the following models of peer support which I use from my own personal lived experience of mental health difficulties and recovery. The ones that relate most to me in my own recovery are as follows: CHIME[1] and Intentional Peer Support. CHIME is an acronym highlighting some of the most significant concepts in mental health recovery: Connection, Hope, Identity, Meaning and Empowerment. This concept helps people communicate in ways outside their current story. Mutuality can be defined as the following: redefining help as a co-learning and growing process so that both parties benefit from the process. In peer support, we encourage one another to re-evaluate how we've come to know what we need to know through the medium of mutuality.

In fostering mutuality in this role I brought my own interpersonal skills to the role and I used active dialogue and open dialogue as well as active listening, trust, empathy and collaboration. I also used strategic sharing of my lived experience to support peers in their recovery. I listened to my peers story and encouraged them to reflect on their feelings and validate them. This built a connection with my peers and created hope and identity. Identity was also built through my presence which served to reduce feelings of isolation and stigma. I paid particular attention to remaining authentic and used open dialogue and an open communicative style.

Peer support is based on the belief that peers who have faced, endured and overcome adversity can offer useful support, encouragement and hope to others facing similar situations. When reciprocity is built it ensures both parties are both givers and receivers. I discussed recovery as a journey from crisis to a place of living well.

As I fostered positive relationships with my peers over a cup of tea in the office a growing relationship was formed and the peer and peer supporter entered a learning process which was beneficial in the development of mutuality. The approaches/skills I used in my practice to build mutuality were the following ones

- Sharing experiences, strategies and stories of hope.
- Encouraging people to take responsibility for their life and recovery.

- Encouraging people without doing things for them.
- Providing people with relevant information.
- Helping people to build their own social networks.
- Supporting people to ensure that their human rights are respected
- Empathetic listening, coaching and being an advocate
- Using active and participatory listening
- Validating feelings and exploring feelings with the person I am supporting
- Peer connection.
- Building hope and identity and strategic sharing of stories.
- Allowing peers to tell their own unique story in their own unique way.
- Facilitating a space for open dialogue
- Being non-judgemental and creating a safe space for the peer.

By practising one-to-one support through strategically sharing my story of mental health difficulties and recovery and authentically listening to the story of my peers I built mutuality on the issues that were important to my fellow peers. Moving forward with the peers at their own pace and supporting them to create their own unique vision of themselves allowed them to find and discover identity and connectivity and allowed them to envisage a process of moving forward towards recovery from mental health difficulties and create a new life full of possibility and hope. In my own lived experience, mutuality and peer support made this possible. It is the very core of what peer support is built on and is what peer support should look like .It is a vital ingredient in the paradigm of peer support and it is in building mutuality through communication and an open communicative style and real conversations that occur in the simplistic sense of the relationship that understanding and personal growth becomes possible. Mutuality fosters hope and empowerment within one's self and is part of the toolbox of life which allows the peer to create a new life for themselves when recovering from mental health difficulties and follow the pathway that leads to recovery. Recovery is thus a journey that has been walked by the peer and peer supporter through lived experience and it is in sharing this journey through mutuality that new horizons and new destinations appear what may have seemed impossible in life now becomes possible as one enters recovery. Mutuality allows a new map of one's life to be created which can be altered at any stage of life and in my own opinion a vital cog on the wheel of peer support which can never be underestimated. In my opinion it is vital in peer support in building relationships with peers and fostering a culture of support, empathy, open communication, trust and positivity. Building mutuality is therefore very significant in peer to peer relationships and in essence essential to peer support.

As Sandra notes here, although the sharing of experiences is a vital component within the principle of mutuality, there are other factors at play. These include the peer's presence and their ability to actively listen. Additionally, other principles are utilised such as reciprocity (see Section 4.2.2) along with other concepts associated with recovery including the wellness toolbox, which forms part of Wellness Recovery Action Planning (WRAP) (Copeland, 2018) and the CHIME model which was created by Leamy et al. (2011) to explain the key aspects of a person's recovery journey.

4.2.2 Reciprocity

Peer support relationships can also be described as reciprocal – where actors involved in the relationship both give and receive facets from each other with the purpose of supporting one another (Davidson et al., 2006; Thiele et al., 2019). At its most basic and purest form, reciprocity is closely linked to mutuality as no individual involved in the relationship can claim expertise, rather both parties work together as equals, share lived experiences and work through problems together to generate solutions that are practical, achievable and ultimately meaningful to both the parties (Repper et al., 2013). This reciprocal nature of peer support has been proven to increase the levels of engagement and improve overall relationship quality between the service user, their assigned peer and their overarching multidisciplinary team (Mullineaux, 2017). An example of reciprocity comes from Nguyen et al., (2022)'s study where a participant spoke on how through creating a mutual environment through the sharing of experiences, the peer also attained fulfilment and empowerment to do their work, as the peers in this study experience of psychosis became a powerful tool that could be used to support others in similar experiences.

4.2.3 Non-Directiveness

Peer support work is not about adding another expert into the room. In fact, peer support work supports people by helping them to recognise their own strengths and resources for recovery (Repper et al., 2013). This is known in the peer support literature as non-directiveness. In the social sciences, non-directiveness refers to a shift in control from service provider to service user where the service user works with the service provider on what they want for their life and their recovery whilst acknowledging the support received by the providers (Johnsen et al., 2017). Within peer support, the goal is always to allow the therapeutic work to be governed and directed by the service user and not the provider (Norton, 2024a). This is essential in peer support work as recovery from mental health is a unique, non-linear process (Anthony, 1993; Erondu and McGraw, 2021). Allowing such work to be self-directed ensures a unique, personalised service which aligns with the service user's hopes, goals, needs and preferences (Norton, 2024a).

4.2.4 Hope

Hope is a concept that has particular relevance in times of crisis leading to a desire to change (Schrank et al., 2011). Yet it is also an important element of mental health recovery (Honey et al., 2023). In terms of this present text, we will utilise Schiavon et al. (2017)'s definition of hope, which is described as a state of positive motivation relating to three essential components: (1) objectives – what goal to achieve, (2) pathways – the plan to achieve the goal and (3) agency – having the motivation towards the objective. Hope as a concept is central to peer support work (Price, 2021). There are a number of reasons for this. Firstly peer support instils hope by demonstrating to the service user that there is light at the end of the tunnel (Barlow et al., 2010). That light involves a sense of meaning and purpose in life beyond mental health difficulties (Rosenberg and Argentzell, 2018). It also involves the normalisation of experiences (Hunt and Byrne, 2019) and the realisation that one is no longer alone and isolated in their battle against mental health difficulties (Mullineaux, 2017). Additionally, the presence of the peer alone is enough to instil hope due to their role-modelling function (Barr et al., 2020). The power of the peer to instigate change noted above is through their own lived experiences of mental health challenges, which is noted as essential for its initiation and sustainability within an individual (Cabral et al., 2014). In our second case study, William explores the principle of hope further and uses it in his own peer support practices with young people in the UK.

Case Study 2:   What is Hope within Peer Support?

William Gallini-Poole

When I first started working with young people, I struggled with where my role was. I was working within a new project, a tier four service[2] with the goal of the project supporting young people in the community, where they would otherwise be admitted to inpatient units. Supporting young people who were incredibly unwell and on the edge of admission was something I hadn't done before – the majority of my work up until that point was systems change and culture shift, so it was an adjustment for myself to find where lived experience suited the project. About a year in, I had raised this with a colleague who had been working in a similar project for many years. During our conversation, they said something that really clicked with me, and guided the way I support the people I work with. They told me that they see themselves as someone who was able to hold the hope for the people and families they work with, where in crisis the families aren't able to. Someone present who had been where they were, and is now living a life worth living. I don't know exactly why, but this really stuck with me as a core principle of the peer support work I do now, even four years later.

To be honest – that quote isn't anything too complicated, but it really struck me. Hope is something I do think some people take for granted – that feeling of aspiration, desire and anticipation for life and what could be. It's also something I didn't have until very recently. Being very unwell as a child, I never had aspirations for life, as I was focusing on being alive day-to-day. For that reason, I do struggle to define hope at times. The more I think about hope as an idea within peer support, the more I settle on just how important it really is. Both for my life and my work as a person now, but also for the recovery journey I've been on for the past five years. But the more I work with mental health, the more I see how quickly that hope vanishes while being unwell. Don't get me wrong, my experiences of being unwell meant I knew this to be the case, but it always saddens me to see just how quickly that hope for life does vanish while being unwell, both for families and the individual who is struggling. For me, seeing this just reiterates how important '*holding that hope*' is, both for families and people I work with. It's where I feel lived experience sits within this specific team, and what I feel passionately about when it comes to working in this project – Being able to hold that hope for the people I work with, supporting families to define a life worth living for themselves, and being able to be a beacon of hope. Proof that there is a way out of mental health, and a future – however that looks for the individual.

A Life Worth Living

In a practical sense – what does holding that hope mean? If hope is a feeling of aspiration and anticipation for what could be, how do I '*hold that hope*' as a Peer Support Worker? While I used working with young people as an example here as it all clicked when I started working in this project, but I do think the most important concept is the same when it comes to working with adults too – '*A Life Worth Living*'. I use this phrase almost daily within my work around recovery education, and I genuinely believe understanding what it meant was a turning point for my life and work. Being able to define what a life worth living without stigma or societal perceptions is incredibly difficult for anyone, let alone someone in crisis. We're raised to have this view of ourselves, an aspiration for the future, for a job, a house, having that taken away leaves a distinct feeling of emptiness from my experience. Having to then re-build what the future looks like, while knowing you can never '*recover*' to who you were before – it took me many years to figure out. When I do visits with people, I always make a point to ask them what life looks like for them in the future. There are so many blocks and barriers when it comes to mental health that I find people generally tend to answer with the path of least resistance, parroting what they've been told.

As I slowly get to know them, I introduce the idea of what '*a life worth living*' looks like for them as an individual – what their hopes for the future are. People generally have very different answers when I ask what does the future hold, compared to what does a life worth living look like. An individual with that sense of hope may have similar answers – whereas people I speak to who are in crisis generally have polar opposite answers or have never considered what a life worth living looks like for them. At the end of my time supporting someone, I will always ask the same two questions again. Generally, I find both answers have changed significantly. To me, that's re-introducing hope to an individual. If someone is able to explain what a life worth living looks like, that's a huge step towards re-introducing hope for the future within an individual. I think introducing this idea is incredibly important when working in peer support.

Being Present – Holding Hope

Sometimes, just being present and talking with someone can re-ignite that sense of hope. Internalised stigma means, for many, a life worth living doesn't feel possible. '*Being unwell has ended my life*' is a quote I hear very often at the start of my time with somebody. Being unwell is incredibly isolating – people don't generally discuss serious mental health in wider society. This meant that there was no examples I could find of people who were unwell like I was – no community to belong in. This meant that the most difficult part of recovery for me was not having a '*path*' I could take – having to define what '*well*' looked like for me. That sense of isolation is overpowering, and incredibly difficult to break. Lived experience is incredibly important here – even if we're not doing anything '*special*' as Peer Support Workers in that moment. Sometimes, by just being present and talking through our experiences, we can start to break that isolation. From my experience, there's no distinct model behind it, there's no intentional use in this example. Even if it doesn't immediately make a difference for someone, just knowing that there is a path towards a future worth enjoying is sometimes enough to make a change. Even if it's just one visit – the impact that can make is huge. I remember a visit I did alongside a professional to a young person who I only ever met once. I didn't discuss too much about myself, I didn't have any '*models*' or '*intentional use*' – from my perspective, I did nothing special. However, what I did mention was that when I was young, I was non-verbal. This young person had never met anyone else who could talk through this with him – the visit ended up being 2 hours of us talking about all the complaints and difficulties we had from being non-verbal as a child. I got an email from him two years later going through everything he had since done in his life, and asking about how to become a Peer Support Worker. That hope had been re-ignited for him, that isolation broken from just one meeting.

Hope for Families

When working into CAMHS[3] teams, I found that the biggest impact I had was talking with families. For many young people I see, the family unit tends to really struggle when a child is unwell. The stigma for a parent is huge, whether that's societal, generational or internal. Many parents feel responsible, guilty and don't see a way out of the crisis. Much of the work I do is talking through with them and showing them there is a path out of mental health – there is a future for their child. Many young people also lash out at parents, as they're people they feel the most comfortable with, and know they will be on their side. The value of peer support here, from my experience, is holding the hope here. Being able to say '*I understand*'. It's offering parents a sense of community and understanding, while also supporting them to advocate for themselves. Many parents I've spoken to don't feel able to live their lives when their child is unwell, which is a huge detriment to their own mental health. Having someone who understands, but also has had similar difficulties tell parents they are allowed to look after themselves and live their own life. This gives hope for family units, hope for the future, which is incredibly important when looking at mental health. Returning a sense of '*normal*' back to a parent or carers life is invaluable for breaking down barriers of hope for the parents, but also guilt for the young people.

Hope through Resources

When trying to create hope for an individual, I find resources are very powerful tools. For someone in crisis, there are many blocks to be able to '*see*' a Peer Support Worker. The anxiety of meeting a new person can be huge and stop many people from receiving support as needed. This is something that all services in mental health face, both clinical and peer support. An action we took to combat that was online resources through our local

Recovery Education Centre. Much of the change and impact I've been able to make for individuals hasn't specifically been working one-on-one with them, but through videos, podcast, webinars among other resources.

From talking with different people within peer support, I tend to see a slight anxiety when I discuss online content. It's a shame, as I've seen first-hand how much impact a 10-minute video can have wider than just individual. Having a library of co-produced content available when people are in crisis is something special – having support at someone's fingertips, being able to access support while at work, without the stigma of attending a '*mental health group*' is something I don't hear discussed as much as I think it should be. One of the biggest concerns I hear from people in my support groups is an anxiety around how to put this into place in their life. They feel supported and part of a community within our peer support groups, but as they re-engage with what the '*real world*' and their future looks like, there's an anxiety around putting things into practice. I often hear about how work-places are unsupportive, don't let an individual put coping strategies into place, or just don't feel like a place an individual can be themselves within. One person I do one-on-one work with has mentioned a few times just how helpful having resources and worksheets available on our website is – she's able to support her own well-being within work, giving her hope that she's able to work full time and live a '*life worth living*' from her own definition. That narrative of '*I'm never going to be able to live independently again*' is much less present within her life – she's able to define her future how she wants to, and has practical steps to achieve these goals. For my perspective, that's inspired hope within her which wouldn't otherwise be present, due to open-access resources. Daily support groups wouldn't fit in to her life – a ten minute video running through her support strategies she recorded does. Inspiring hope doesn't just have to be direct contact – it can be one video from many years ago.

William here points to many mechanisms whereby lived experience can be used to instil hope. A lot of these examples are simple but extremely beneficial for the person William is working with. The simplicity of his presence alone, along with the sharing of a similar experience, is enough to instil hope in an individual. William notes how instilling hope in the family is also a necessary function as they have their own journey to follow and it is ok for them to look after themselves (Norton and Cuskelly, 2021). Also of note in this case study is the acknowledgement that instilling hope is not a one-time, static procedure. In fact, peers at times must hold and nurture the person's hope until they are able to be reacquainted.

4.2.5 Strengths-Based

Peer support work should be strengths-based in their clinical approach to service users (Berry et al., 2011). Essentially, strengths-based in the context of the peer refers to the intentional focus on a person's capabilities and abilities rather than their deficits, so that the individual develops the confidence required to embark on their own unique recovery journey and make strides towards recovery (Xie, 2013). As a result, the therapeutic power of the approach is its overt bias towards a person's strengths (Rapp and Sullivan, 2014), as it is through this focus that individuals start to uncover their own abilities, take personal responsibility for their life and recovery journey and make positive strides towards wellness. Peers should view the person they work with by their strengths from the very first meeting where their personal narrative/story of recovery is shared. Essentially the narrative is the first attempt by the peer to work in a strengths-focused manner as the narrative is partially utilised here as a tool to demonstrate the peer's strengths attributed to them by their lived experiences of mental health challenges (Pattoni, 2012).

4.2.6 Inclusive

Being a peer is more than just the experience of having a mental health challenge; rather it is about the meaning and understanding one gets from such experiences (Repper et al., 2013). This can be difficult if one comes from a marginalised community. In addition, Peer Support Workers do strive towards destigmatisation, eradicating discrimination and prejudice against an individual on the basis of whether or not they have a mental health challenge (Health Service Executive, n.d.). This idea of inclusion, regardless of creed or difficulty, is slowly becoming a component of peer support with colleges like Atlantic Technological University in the west of Ireland providing a peer training course that allows one to specialise in a certain area often considered marginalised to the general population, for example neurodiversity (Atlantic Technological University, 2022). This sense of inclusion is also becoming evident theoretically with the literature on peer support for marginalised populations ever increasing (Mahon, 2023; Chikezie, 2024; Harty, 2024; O'Donnell and Cusack, 2024; Wright and Mahon, 2024; Usideme, 2024).

4.2.7 Progressive

Peer support work is not about creating a *'friendship'* that is static (Repper et al., 2013), instead it is a *'friend like'* relationship that is intentional in that it has a purpose. As we will discover in later chapters (Chapters 7 and 8), the purpose of the role is to break down barriers to create a state known as informality, which by its very nature the relationship transforms into something 'friend like' (Norton, 2022). This informality is important for the creation of a genuine relationship based on the peer principles we have been discussing thus far. However, as Chapter 8 specifically highlights, this brings with it ethical dilemmas within the relationship, particularly towards the emotional safety of both parties involved (Norton, 2023). However, when carefully managed, the peer and service user can go on a shared journey of discovery where they both learn new skills, develop new resources and re-examine challenges to find workable solutions (Repper et al., 2013).

4.2.8 Safe

Indeed as per the discussion in Section 4.2.7, to create informality safely, both parties need to understand what emotional safety means to them and then nego-tiate with one another to develop a shared understanding of safety (Repper et al., 2013). This often occurs through the formalised aspects of the peer role, particu-larly when working in statutory bodies like the Irish health services. Such areas for discussion include the times of the day when a peer can safely take the call from a service user, use equipment that belongs to statutory services and not the individual peer, and boundaries in terms of when to meet and how to connect with each other – both through social media and/or other methods of telecommunica-tion. An example of guidance regarding safety comes from the Health Service Executive (2020) when guidelines were developed to ensure peer support contin-ued safely despite the systematic and global disruption that occurred as a result of the Covid-19 pandemic.

4.2.9 Values and Competencies of Peer Support Work

In addition to the above central principles, there are a number of values and associ-ated competencies attached to peer support. Again, this is a non-exhaustive list but represents the most common values and competencies within the literature. The first set of values and competencies come from Intentional Peer Support, which was originally developed by Shery Mead in the USA during the 1990s (Intentional Peer Support, 2024). Within the same, a number of values and associated compe-tencies regarding peer support work in mental health have been identified (Mead, 2014) (see Table 4.1). Each of these values and associated competencies link back to one of the eight foundational principles of peer support noted above, but the wording is based solely on the creator of the approach for Intentional Peer Support (IPS).

As one can notice, as peer support work has grown in terms of formality, so too has the number of attempts to define and describe these values (Watson, 2019). Take for instance the current example from Mead's Intentional Peer Support. In the

Table 4.1 Intentional Peer Support Values and Associated Competencies

No.	Value	Competency
1	**Commitment to recovery, growth, evolution and inspiring hope**	• Demonstrates willingness to challenge self, others and the relationship. • Demonstrates the intention of learning as opposed to the intention of helping.
2	**Accountability (Personal and Relational)**	• Follow through with commitments. • Attends and fully participates in co-supervision. • Continues to become accomplished in IPS skills.
3	**The power of language**	• Has awareness of the power of language. • Uses language that is free of jargon, assumptions, judgements, generalizations and characterizations (e.g. medical language).
4	**Direct honest respectful communication**	• Awareness of own intentions (e.g. agendas, assumptions). • Is authentic. • Values and validates others. • Gives and receives difficult messages with awareness of other worldviews. • Ability to communicate in a way that invites sharing of perspectives.
5	**Consciousness raising/critical learning**	• Desire and ability to self-reflect. • Demonstrates an understanding of how people can get stuck in a "mental patient" role. • Uses personal self-awareness to stimulate growth in others.
6	**Worldview, diversity, holding multiple truths, trauma-informed.**	• Demonstrates an understanding of how people's past experiences impact who they are, how they think, how they relate etc. • Awareness of when personal strong beliefs cut off other's "truths". • Ability to self-reflect.
7	**Mutual responsibility and belief in the power of relationship.**	• Maintains awareness of power and privilege. • Focuses on the relationship and whether it is working for both parties. • Is able to state observations, acknowledge own feelings, and request what is needed for the relationship to work. • Is able to see and "own" their part of a conflict.

Table 4.1 (Continued)

No.	Value	Competency
8	**Shared risk.**	• Ability to demonstrate sitting with discomfort. • Ability to negotiate fear/anger/conflict. • Ability to avoid overreacting and taking over even when things get tough (e.g. being mindful of power, mutuality and personal accountability).
9	**Moving towards.**	• Demonstrates an ability to distinguish between moving towards something positive and moving away from something negative. • Invites conversation that shifts problem-focus to creating-focus.
10	**Creating community and social change.**	• Demonstrates IPS in all relationships and actions. • Draws on people's interests outside peer support. • Has familiarity with local resources. • Supports people in finding and trying new community resources. • Advocates for people to address mental health challenges in the context of community relationships.

Source: Adopted From Mead (2014).

ten years since the identification of the original values and corresponding competencies, in 2024, these same competencies identified in Mead (2014) were adapted to represent newfound evidence (Table 4.2). However, along with these changes, Mead (2019) has also developed a self-assessment tool that allows intentional peers to assess their alignment with these competencies within their own, individual peer support practice. The 2024 version of this self-assessment tool is reproduced in Table 4.2

.The Substance Abuse and Mental Health Services Administration [SAMHSA] adds to Mead's work by suggesting a number of core competencies of peer support work. These core competencies and their associated categories were generated through co-production and consensus with members of both the mental health and substance use recovery communities, including service users of these communities, and are outlined in Table 4.3 (SAMHSA, n.d., 2015).

Table 4.2 Intentional Peer Support Core Competencies Self-Assessment Tool

Competency 1	Connection: Nurtures and Cultivates Connection with Others
Description	Demonstrates warmth, openness, curiosity and interest in others' experiences, stories and perspectives • Pays attention to where we connect and what we have in common, versus getting side-tracked by differences or dislikes. • Is aware of disconnection • Reconnects with authenticity, owning one's own part

Rating Scale	1	2	3	4	5
	Unaware of impact on relationship of valuing or validating responses.	Some attention to impact on relationship of valuing and validation.	Intermittent attention to impact on relationship of valuing and validation.	Frequent attention to impact on relationship of impact of valuing and validation	Continual awareness of impact on relationship of valuing and validation

Competency 2	Shifting the Focus from Helping to Learning Together
Description	• Sees others as capable co-learners and responsible adults; does not take an advising or problem-solving role • Approaches relationship with curiosity and interest (versus set ideas, assumptions and predictions) • Hears what can be learned from someone else's way of looking at things rather than imposing their own viewpoint • Is open to new ideas and ways of seeing things

Rating Scale	1	2	3	4	5
	Usually assumes the role of helper, with little effort to learn from or about the other.	Makes some effort to learn with others, but usually begins with or shifts into helping.	Combines helping and learning in approximately equal measure.	Primarily learning with each other, but occasionally shifts into helping.	Nearly always learning from each other.

(Continued)

Table 4.2 (Continued)

Competency 3	Worldview: Awareness of Own and Other's Worldview
Description	• Understands that 'worldview' is the way we see the world based on our own experiences • Is aware of own worldview and readily explores own assumptions • Is comfortable with exploring and affirming others' worldviews, listening with curiosity for the untold story • Understands that trauma-awareness means listening for 'what happened' rather than for 'what's wrong' • Uses language that explores meaning rather than diagnosis or symptom language

Rating Scale	1	2	3	4	5
	Unconscious of worldview. Nearly always takes own and other's told story at face value. Worldview differences are seen as 'right or wrong'	Developing awareness of differences in worldview. Conversation stays mostly on the surface. Feels that some worldviews are clearly better than others.	Conscious of worldview. Starting to explore and open up untold stories. Still responds from a place of 'knowing', but beginning to acknowledge alternate perspectives	Consciously exploring worldview and opening up the untold story. No longer presumes to know others' experiences or have answers for them. Invites and respects alternate perspectives.	Exploration of worldview and untold story are integrated natural responses. Do not make assumptions about others' experiences. Demonstrates deep respect and appreciation of multiple perspectives.

Competency 4	Shifting the Focus from the Individual to the Relationship
Description	• Works to co-create relationships that work well for all concerned • Notices disconnections, and is prepared to explore assumptions, patterns, power/privilege, and meaning • Invites and encourages feedback about how the relationship is working for all parties concerned

Rating Scale	1	2	3	4	5
	Gives little or no attention to relationship; almost entirely focused on individuals and their needs	Demonstrates some awareness of relationship and the need to nurture the relationship, although the interaction is focused on individual needs	Touches on relationship and nurturing the relationship in conversation, but focus is still on individual needs and concerns	Attends to relationship and the need to nurture it directly in conversation, but may occasionally overlook this when it is relevant	Continually aware of relationship; addresses need to nurture relationship both pro-actively and spontaneously in a way that deepens mutual understanding and connection.

(Continued)

Table 4.2 (Continued)

Competency 5	Mutuality

Description	• Actively invites and makes space for everyone's perspectives without either ignoring others or imposing
	• Negotiates relational needs and interests in ways that work for everyone (self as well as others)
	• Seeks to negotiate power and privilege in ways that work for everyone
	  ○ Is aware of and able to own power and privilege held by self and others
	  ○ Invites mutual exploration of the impact on the relationship
	• Works to share risk and responsibility rather than taking control

Rating Scale	1	2	3	4	5
	No apparent attention to creating relationships that work for everyone. Needs and interests are ignored or unilaterally asserted with little attempt at negotiation	Beginning awareness of mutuality and shared responsibility. Relationship negotiations remain infrequent and inconsistent. Needs and interests are mostly ignored or unilaterally asserted	Aware of mutuality and shared responsibility. Relationship negotiations seek to address everyone's needs and interests, though genuine co-creation is often lacking	Importance of mutuality and shared responsibility is fully appreciated. Genuine dialogue is invited to negotiate relational needs and interests	Practice of mutuality and shared responsibility appears natural and organic. Relationships are negotiated in ways that appear both co-creative and inspired.

Competency 6	Shifting the focus from fear to hope and possibility

Description	• Forms hope-based relationships, focused on:
	  ○ What is possible
	  ○ Where we are going
	  ○ How we can co-create something new

Rating Scale	1	2	3	4	5
	Focuses almost entirely on 'illness' and managing symptoms. Routinely imposes fear-based concerns on others.	Fear-focused, but able to recognize some fear-based assumptions when they are pointed out.	Sometimes able to see fear-based assumptions on my own, and usually if pointed out. Sometimes able to shift focus to hope and possibility on my own initiative.	Often able to focus on hope and possibility independently. Usually aware of own fears. Sometimes able to self-correct after imposing their own fears on others	Nearly always focuses on exploring possibilities. Aware of and owns personal fears as limited by life experience

(Continued)

Table 4.2 (Continued)

Competency 7	Task 4: Moving towards versus moving away from
Description	• Invites mutual sharing around values, hopes, dreams, possibilities and aspirations for living • Focuses on what is possible rather than what is bad, wrong or isn't wanted • Co-creating rather than focusing on goals or problem-solving

Rating Scale	1	2	3	4	5
	Focuses on moving away from problems, problem-solving and individual goals	Some awareness of possibility, but still focuses on problem-solving and individual solutions	Invites moving toward what is wanted. Sometimes uses problem-solving language.	Consistently invites moving toward what is wanted, co-creating a focus on the relationship-creating focus	Possibilities evolve naturally from the conversation.

Competency 8	Self-Reflection

Description	• Actively reflects on the experience of self in a relationship – able to 'own one's own part'
	• Is aware of own worldview and how it developed, including personal feelings, thoughts, attitudes, assumptions, judgements, agendas, power, privilege, defaults and patterns
	• Welcomes differences in experiences/perspectives/beliefs/judgements as opportunities to learn and grow
	• Resists the tendency to blame others for uncomfortable feelings
	  ○ Uses relational differences or discomfort proactively to notice and examine personal agendas, patterns, default responses and worldview assumptions
	  ○ Asks and explores with curiosity and interest: 'What is my part?'
	  ○ Invites and encourages others to share alternate perspectives and experiences that challenge personal agendas and worldview assumptions
	• Uses self-awareness to build connection by being transparent, approachable and authentic

Rating Scale	1	2	3	4	5
	Unaware of, or not interested in, how own values and assumptions affect relational interactions.	Shows some recognition of own values and assumptions but continues to impose them on others.	Generally able to identify own values and assumptions. Mixed success in refraining from imposing these on others.	Aware of, and willing to own, values and assumptions. Avoids imposing them on others. Able to acknowledge and self-correct as needed.	Deep awareness of own values and assumptions. Uses self-disclosure and transparency to further mutual exploration and relational connection

(Continued)

Table 4.2 (Continued)

Competency 9	Able to Give and Receive Feedback
Description	• Ensures connection • Acknowledges and appreciates others' positive contributions • Looks at the situation through the lens of the other person's life experience, in addition to one's own • Considers whether own worldview is a reflection of privilege or bias • Frames feedback around observation rather than judgement • Keeps the focus on moving towards what is wanted for the relationship (closeness, connection, trust), rather than away from what isn't wanted (dishonesty, dirty dishes) • Invites and gives honest responses • Validates other's responses and demonstrates willingness to learn and be changed by what they have

Rating Scale	1	2	3	4	5
	Fails to allow space for others' experience or consider 'own part' when receiving feedback or difficult messages	Makes some effort to acknowledge others' experience or 'own part' when receiving feedback or difficult messages	Both acknowledges others' experience and 'own part' when receiving feedback or difficult messages. The conversation takes on an appreciably mutual tone	Others' experiences and own part are fully acknowledged. A deeper understanding is actively sought. Mutual learning is apparent.	Receives feedback in a way that naturally deepens relational connection. Validates others' experience, acknowledges own part and opens the door to mutual growth.

Competency 10	Co-Reflection
Description	• Attends co-supervision regularly • Shows up prepared and on time • Readily identifies areas for personal learning and growth • Expresses curiosity about others' intentions and aspirations for co-learning • Maintains connection, mutuality and actively cares for relationships with co-participants • Listens to worldview and explores power and privilege and their impact • Maintains attitudes of hope, possibility, co-learning, co-creation and moving toward during the co-reflection period

Rating Scale	1	2	3	4	5
	No observable commitment to co-supervision. Rarely attends or gets stuck in blaming or fixing	Some observable commitment to co-reflection; demonstrates some willingness to grow in relationships	Observable commitment to co-reflection. Attends regularly and demonstrates a clear interest in relational growth.	Actively participates and uses co-reflection to deepen understanding of – and connection with – self and others	Participates in co-reflection that inspires mutual growth, connection and understanding.

Table 4.3 SAMHSA's Categories and Competencies of Peer Support Work

No.	Category	Context	Competencies
1	Engages peers in collaborative and caring relationships.	Emphasises peer's ability to initiate and develop ongoing relationships.	Initiates contact with peers.
			Listen to peers with careful attention to the content and emotions being communicated.
			Reaches out to engage peers across the whole recovery process/continuum.
			Demonstrate genuine acceptance and respect.
			Demonstrates understanding of peers' experiences and feelings.
2	Provides support.	The peer's ability to provide mutual support.	Values the experiences and feelings of peers.
			Encourages the exploration and pursuit of community roles.
			Conveys hope to peers about their own recovery.
			Celebrates peer's efforts and accomplishments.
			Provides concrete assistance to help peers accomplish goals and tasks.
3	Shares lived experiences of recovery.	Peers need to skilfully utilise their lived experience in a way that inspires and supports a person with mental health challenges.	Relates their own lived experience narrative, and with permission utilise this and the recovery stories of others to inspire hope.
			Discuss ongoing personal efforts to enhance recovery.
			Recognise when to share and when to listen.
			Describe personal recovery practices and support others in discovering recovery practices that work for them.

Table 4.3 (Continued)

No.	Category	Context	Competencies
4	Personalise peer support.	Tailor and individualise peer support provided to peers, in so doing identifying multiple pathways to recovery	Understand personal values and culture and how these contribute to personal biases, beliefs and judgements.
			Respect the cultural and spiritual beliefs and practices of those peers work with.
			Recognise and respond appropriately to the fact that each person has a unique and complex recovery journey to follow.
			Tailor peer support to meet personal preferences and the unique needs of service users/family members.
5	Supports recovery planning.	Support service users/family members to create a recovery plan noting their goals as they relate to home, work, community and health and support them in achieving same.	Support peers in setting goals and dreams for the future.
			Propose mechanisms that will support peers in attaining these goals.
			Support peers to use decision-making strategies when choosing supports and services.
			Help peers to function as part of their multi-disciplinary team.
			Identify credible information from various resources as required.
6	Links to resources, services, and supports.	Help service users/family members acquire resources, services and supports they need to enhance recovery.	Keep up-to-date on community resources and services.
			Assist service users/family members in investigating, selecting and using resources and services.
			Accompany and participate with peers in community activities and appointments as required.

(Continued)

Table 4.3 (Continued)

No.	Category	Context	Competencies
7	Provides information about skills related to health, wellness, and recovery.	Describes how peers coach, model and provide information and skills to enhance recovery.	Educate service users/family members on health, wellness, recovery and related activities.
			Participate alongside service users/family members in co-learning and other enhancing recovery experiences.
			Coach service users/family members on how to access treatments, services, and how to navigate the system.
			Coach individuals in desired skills and strategies.
			Educate supporters regarding recovery and related supports.
			Utilise approaches that match the preferences and needs of the service user/family member.
8	Help peers manage crises.	Identify risks and use mechanisms to reduce risk to service users and others.	Recognise signs of distress and threats to personal integrity and their environment.
			Provide reassurance.
			Create safe spaces when meeting service users/family members.
			Take action to address distress by using knowledge of local resources as well as the preference of the service user.
			Assist in the development of advanced directives and other crisis prevention tools.
9	Values communication.	How peers interact verbally and in writing with colleagues and others.	Use respectful, person-centred written and verbal language when interacting with the service user, their family, community and others.

Table 4.3 (Continued)

No.	Category	Context	Competencies
			Actively listen.
			Clarify their understanding of information to relieve doubt regarding meaning.
			Convey service user/family member's point of view when working with colleagues.
			Document information in accordance with local policy and procedures.
			Comply with rules regarding confidentiality and the person's right to privacy.
10	Support collaboration and teamwork.	Develop and maintain effective relationships with colleagues and others	Work with colleagues to enhance the provision off services.
			Engage providers from different specialities to meet the needs of the service users.
			Partner with others to strengthen opportunities of the peer.
			Strive to resolve conflicts in relationships with service users/family members and other support networks
11	Promote leadership and advocacy.	Describes actions that support peers to provide leadership in advancing a recovery-orientated mission for services. In addition, advocate for the legal and human rights of the service user/family member.	Use knowledge of relevant legislation and rights to ensure the rights of the service user/family member are respected.
			Advocate for the needs and desires of the service user/family member.
			Participate in efforts to reduce and eliminate prejudice and discrimination.
			Educate colleagues on recovery and the use of recovery supports.

(Continued)

Table 4.3 (Continued)

No.	Category	Context	Competencies
			Participate in efforts to improve the organisation.
			Maintain a positive peer/professional reputation with relevant communities.
12	Promotes growth and development	Becoming a more reflective practitioner who is professional and competent in their practice.	Recognise one's own limits in terms of knowledge and seek assistance from others as required.
			Use supervision effectively by monitoring self, preparing adequately before meetings, and engaging in problem-solving with supervisors.
			Reflect on personal motivations and feelings associated with peer work, recognising distress and knowing when to seek support.
			Seek opportunities to increase knowledge and skills of peer support.

Source: Adapted from SAMHSA (2015).

In addition in 2017, ENRICH, a programme of research led by Steve Gillard and colleagues to create fidelity criteria for peer support work, created five key principles which mental health services that are based upon/or include peer support should follow (Figure 4.1) (Gillard et al., 2017). These principles include the following:

1. Build safe and trusting relationships based on shared lived experience.
2. Ensure that principles of mutuality and reciprocity underpin all peer support relationships.
3. Promote the application and validation of experiential knowledge (see Chapter 6) in peer support.
4. Enable leadership in how peer support is given and received.
5. Enable peers to discover their own strengths and to build and strengthen connections to other peers and wider society.

(Gillard et al., 2017)

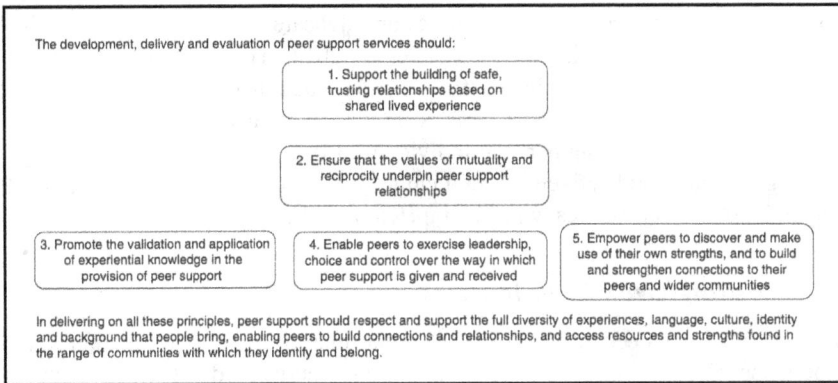

The development, delivery and evaluation of peer support services should:

1. Support the building of safe, trusting relationships based on shared lived experience

2. Ensure that the values of mutuality and reciprocity underpin peer support relationships

3. Promote the validation and application of experiential knowledge in the provision of peer support

4. Enable peers to exercise leadership, choice and control over the way in which peer support is given and received

5. Empower peers to discover and make use of their own strengths, and to build and strengthen connections to their peers and wider communities

In delivering on all these principles, peer support should respect and support the full diversity of experiences, language, culture, identity and background that people bring, enabling peers to build connections and relationships, and access resources and strengths found in the range of communities with which they identify and belong.

Figure 4.1 The ENRICH Peer Support Principles.

Gillard and colleagues studied this in their 2021 publication where they utilised these principles to co-construct fidelity criteria for services. Although these criteria will not be discussed within this text, it is a useful tool to examine service readiness for Peer Support Workers within traditional mental health services.

4.3 Roles of the Peer Support Worker

Like the principles/values of peer support, the roles of this group of mental health practitioners are extensive, which has led to a lack of role clarity within peer support work (Janouskova et al., 2022; Krumm et al., 2022; Adams et al., 2023). Another rationale for this lack of role clarity is the peer's role overlaps with other professional roles on the MDT (Moll et al., 2009; Mayer and McKenzie, 2017). However, it has since been established that they apply such roles using a different knowledge set – that of experiential knowledge, which will be discussed further in Chapter 6 of this book (Norton, 2024b). Regardless, such lack of clarity remains, and as such, the remainder of this chapter is dedicated to highlighting the major roles and responsibilities of the peer. It is important to note here that this is not a non-exhaustive list of roles as the very nature of peer means the interplay of many different roles that may fall into certain other specialities but are applied through the central knowledge set attributed to lived experience (Norton, 2024b). To support the discussion regarding roles, a sample job specifications document has been attached to this chapter as an appendix to further document the variety of roles the peer possess to do their work (see Appendix]. The most pertinent roles and responsibilities are now outlined below.

4.3.1 Advocacy

Advocacy in peer support refers to the support provided to the service user to either speak for themselves or if requested, and with the permission of the party, speak on their behalf (South Eastern Health and Social Care Trust, n.d.). In peer support work, the Peer Support Worker can act as an advocate for the service users they are supporting (Berry et al., 2011; Cabral et al., 2014). However, as we will later uncover in Chapter 7 of this book, it is recommended that this process occurs at the start of the peer relationship. This is important because the ultimate goal of peer support work is to support the individual in identifying their own strengths, building new ones and actively using them to live a life of their own choice (NHS England, 2023; Peer Advocacy in Mental Health, n.d.).

4.3.2 Sharing Lived Experience

A key role of the Peer Support Worker is the therapeutic sharing of their lived experience (Cabral et al., 2014; Health Service Executive, n.d.). This lived experience, as we will discover further in Chapter 6, is a yet to be fully recognised knowledge set known as experiential knowledge (Norton, 2023). It works by helping the peer to connect with service users on a human level and in doing so provides hope to these individuals that recovery from mental health challenges is possible (Cabral et al., 2014). It is also an important component in the creation of informality, which as we will learn in Chapter 7 is key to allowing the individual the time, space and ability to look at what they want from life and putting provisions in place to achieve these goals together (Norton, 2022). However, there is a continuous debate regarding how the peer should share their lived experience of distress and recovery with an individual. For instance, should the peer share the entire narrative or story of recovery or just what is similar to the individual they are working with (Bailie, 2015; Mulluneaux, 2017; Kumar et al., 2019)? Olga adds to this debate in Case Study 3, where she highlights the continuous nature of this debate even in her work as a peer delivering recovery education in the UK.

Case Study 3:   The Role of Lived Experience in Peer Support Work: Insights from a Peer Worker Acting as a Recovery College Facilitator

Olga Zilberberg

Peer support is a form of social support where individuals with similar experiences, provide emotional, social, and practical assistance to each other. Unlike traditional therapeutic relationships, peer support is built on mutuality, shared experience, and a sense of equality. Peer support plays a vital role in mental health recovery, since peer supporters have faced similar struggles, they offer a level of understanding that is often deeply meaningful to others in recovery. Research from the field of mental health peer support shows that disclosing lived experience helps normalise conversations about mental health. The more people share, the more the stigma surrounding mental illness diminishes, fostering a culture of openness and empathy. Sharing experiences within Recovery College settings is part of the journey that both students and peers go through. Recovery colleges take an educational, rather than a therapeutic approach to equip people through a variety of recovery-focused courses with the knowledge, understanding and practical skills to best manage their mental well-being.

The ethos of Recovery Colleges is to convey messages of hope, empowerment, possibility and aspiration, none of which could be achieved without the power sharing of lived experiences in a non-judgemental space. In Recovery colleges individuals are encouraged to explore ways to express their challenges in a manner that fosters self-discovery and self-reflection. When sharing experiences, every individual works towards carefully crafting their own narrative to provide new perspectives to others around mental illness, thereby increasing hope and promoting flexible thinking. The group always provides a sense of community, and their understanding creates a sense of psychological safety in which everyone is welcome to openly support.

The way experiences are shared is varied. There are countless number of opportunities available for individuals to support each other and for peers to 'intervene' when self-disclosure is needed to increase self-empowerment of individuals. Such opportunities are – guided group discussions during sessions and with the focus on a particular topic – hope, motivation, strengths, courage, recovery journey. Casual conversations can also take place during tea and coffee breaks when students, facilitators and peers gather around to reflect on the learnings or to expand on a topic discussed during the session in a less formal environment. In some areas where Recovery Colleges have a physical site, students can visit the office to book onto new courses or ask for advice on which step they could take next. In such situation, staff members or peers work with individuals on drafting Individual Learning Plans that allow students to explore and plan their learning, their journey and set up goals. In such instances, students tend to open up about their challenges and difficulties. Peer Support Worker, peer volunteers and staff members empathies and validate the students' challenges sharing their own lived experiences, how they might have overcome some of them and what they learnt along the way.

In my many years of working in Recovery Colleges, I have noticed that the outcome of sharing lived experiences is inspiration. When individuals share their challenges and how they overcame them in a positive way, they create a ripple effect that sets mental health recovery in motion. It is extremely rewarding to see how individuals inspire each other. The power of sharing lived experiences in mental health peer support plays a dual role – offering benefits to both the individual receiving support and the one providing it. Research highlights the therapeutic impact of storytelling and peer disclosure, emphasising that sharing can be empowering and validating. For the individual recovering from mental health challenges, hearing someone else's story can reduce feelings of isolation, foster hope, and provide practical insights for coping. The peer supporter, by sharing their lived experience, can gain a sense of purpose, deepen their understanding of their own recovery journey, and contribute to dismantling stigma.

Additionally, studies such as those by the National Institute for Health Research (NIHR) have highlighted the cathartic benefits of disclosing personal experiences. Peer supporters often report feeling a sense of emotional release, self-acceptance, and validation when they share their recovery stories. This act of vulnerability also enhances their own reflective practices, helping them to recognise how far they've come in their recovery. However, while disclosure can be therapeutic, there are potential emotional risks for the peer supporter, especially when reliving traumatic experiences. Without proper support mechanisms, repeated disclosure can lead to emotional fatigue or even vicarious trauma. Thus, sharing lived experiences needs to be done with caution. Self-disclosure can compromise rapport building and connection if the information shared is not relevant, overburdens or overwhelms others around. As peer supporters, we need to be mindful of how much details we give of our own experience so that we remain professional and helpful in our role. Oversharing information can create role confusion in terms of students feeling that they need to support the peer worker in their struggles or students not wanting to disclose their own challenges not to add more distress onto the peer worker.

Safeguarding oneself plays a key part on how helpful we can be in our interactions with others. Self-disclosure of lived experience needs to be measured and carefully thought so that it does not jeopardise the well-being of the peer worker. We need to be aware that talking about our own experience can trigger us and stir emotions in us that we might find hard to deal with. Therefore, being able to pause and ask ourselves what we are about to disclose and for what purpose is a useful strategy to measure our words. Ethical considerations are at the heart of effective mental health peer support, ensuring that both the peer supporter and those they assist are protected from potential harm. Peer supporters must carefully navigate the balance between the therapeutic benefits of self-disclosure and the risks of oversharing. Therefore, it is essential for peer supporters to reflect on what they choose to disclose, ensuring that it serves the purpose of support and does not overwhelm or detract from the recovery process. If disclosure serves the purpose of building rapport, encouraging action, increasing hope, to normalising or validating the person's feelings or experiences or offering a new perspective, as some examples, then I can take a step back and ask myself: how much do I need to disclose and what words would I use?

So, how can we protect ourselves and maintain our well-being?

Protecting oneself from the effects of others' sharing their stories with us is crucial as well as having self-awareness of when we are processing internal emotions that have raised from us sharing our own stories. To mitigate these risks, peer supporters must prioritise the SELF. Evidence-based guidelines suggest several protective strategies, such as the use of supervision, support networks or peers' forums, boundary setting and training and education. It is paramount that peer supporters set clear boundaries- both emotional and professional boundaries, so they avoid compassion fatigue, burnout and being retraumatised by others' challenges. Emotional and professional boundaries help create a safe and structured environment for both the peer supporter and the person they are helping, ensuring that the *helping relationship* remains healthy and productive. Emotional boundaries allow the peer supporter to remain empathetic and engaged without becoming overly absorbed in the other person's struggles. By maintaining a clear distinction between their own emotional state and the challenges of those they support, peer supporters can prevent emotional exhaustion. This separation helps protect them from being overwhelmed by difficult emotions or becoming retraumatised by the stories they hear.

Professional boundaries, on the other hand, ensure that the peer supporter maintains their role as a facilitator of support, rather than becoming overextended by taking on more responsibility than is appropriate. This means respecting the limitations of their position, understanding when to refer someone to a professional, and recognising that their role is to offer empathy and shared experience, not to provide therapeutic intervention. Boundaries create a framework that allows both parties to engage meaningfully without overstepping into areas that could cause harm. For the peer supporter, this structure also helps in managing the emotional intensity of the work, reducing the risk of burnout and fostering long-term sustainability in their role. We cannot underestimate the importance of structured support systems for peer supporters. Engaging in regular supervision and reflective practice allows the peer supporters to debrief and process their experiences, ensuring they do not become overwhelmed by what they share.

Supervision, in particular, serves as a formal space for peer supporters to reflect on their experiences, discuss challenges, and receive guidance on maintaining boundaries. Regular supervision not only helps them process any emotional strain but also ensures that they are adhering to best practices in their supporting roles. Reflective practice within these sessions allows for deep introspection, helping peer supporters to understand their own emotional responses, build resilience, and avoid becoming overwhelmed by the emotional content of their work. Some Recovery Colleges offer a multi-tiered support system, with quarterly supervision, monthly peer forums, and weekly informal chats. Peer supporters find that this system offers multiple avenues to debrief depending on the immediacy of their needs and balance between formal and informal support.

Finally, through education and training Peer Support Workers can cultivate self-awareness, to recognise early signs of emotional strain and pro-actively engage in self-care practices such as mindfulness, exercise, or simply taking time to recharge. Regularly reflecting on their emotional state allows them to maintain their own mental well-being, ensuring they can continue to offer effective support without compromising their health. Prioritising self-care not only prevents burnout but also models healthy coping strategies for those they support, reinforcing the importance of balance and emotional resilience in recovery.

In conclusion, peer support is a transformative component of mental health recovery and the use of lived experience in peer support is a powerful tool that, when used thoughtfully, enhances the effectiveness of mental health support. However, for peer supporters to be effective in sharing personal experiences, sharing needs to be done in a careful and purposeful way to foster connection, inspire hope, and contribute meaningfully to the recovery journey of those they support, all while safeguarding their own well-being. Peers must practice self-care, maintain emotional and professional boundaries, and utilise structured support systems like supervision and reflective practice to safeguard their well-being, continue to provide effective support and help create a culture of openness and empowerment within the Recovery College.

As noted by Olga, there is no solid approach to sharing lived experiences. It seems to be a personal decision as to what is shared and when and how it is shared. However, Olga also notes the potential implications, particularly to the Peer Support Worker's own well-being in sharing such experiences. This includes the risk of emotional vulnerability and distress within the peer relationship. This will be discussed further as part of our discussions regarding the ethical dilemmas of peer support in Chapter 8. However, it is important to share at this stage that sharing lived experiences is a risky business that individual peers need to be aware of so that when they do share, it does not end up becoming a source of vulnerability and unwellness for the individual.

4.3.3 Recovery Champion/Role Modelling

Peer Support Workers are considered role models of recovery (Viking et al., 2022). Not just for the service user undergoing their own recovery journey, but also from within the system where they are considered champions of recovery within the said service. Within their role-modelling capacity, this role is directly linked to the peer support principle of hope (as discussed above) as it is through this role-modelling function that hope for a positive future in recovery is instilled within these individuals (Krumm et al., 2022). This role model functionality is also used to convince traditional staff that peers can be professional within services and with those that they come into contact with over the course of their work (Skills for Health, n.d.). In this way, the role-modelling functionality of the peer is multi-directional as it not only impacts those the peer is working with but also other members of the multi-disciplinary team as well (The Housing Agency, n.d.).

4.3.4 Re-Integration into the Community

After the knowledge associated with lived experience, knowledge as it pertains to what resources are out there in the local community to support recovery is the next most important function of the peer in mental health service provision. The peer in this situation acts as a bridge between the service user/family member and their wider community. The peer, by virtue of discovering this through their own recovery journey, is often described as having '*insider*' knowledge of their local communities (Panaite et al., 2024). As a result, this supports the rationale for peers in traditional services to be placed mainly on community-based multi-disciplinary teams as this is where the peer can have the most impact in the rehabilitation of the individual towards meaningful roles within their wider community (Heon, 2024). Such rehabilitation cannot occur in isolation. As such, rehabilitation through connection with community resources is imperative to the treatment regimens of those engaging in peer support in the community (Cha et al., 2024).

4.3.5 Mediator

As noted above, it is well documented that the Peer Support Worker functions as a bridge between the service user and provider due to the tenuous position they hold as both professional and friend (see Chapters 7 and 8) (Gillard et al., 2014; Lennox et al., 2021). Given this intersectionality of positions, the peer is required to be able to negotiate and mediate on behalf of the service user (Health Service Executive, n.d.). Indeed the peer's role in wider conflict management within multi-disciplinary teams is being increasingly realised due to their ability to relate, access and foster understanding between both parties concerned (The Workplace Mediation, 2023). This role is important as it is seen as vital in narrowing the '*them vs us*' gap still evident between staff and the service users/family members they serve today (Walde et al., 2023).

4.4 Concluding Remarks

This chapter aimed to explore the principles, values and roles of the Peer Support Worker in mental health service provision. Through the support of three case studies, this chapter identified eight principles, five roles and a number of values of peer support working in mental health. These are by no means exhaustive but do in fact reflect the most important principles, values and roles of the peer at the time of writing (2024). The next chapter of this text further adds to the discussions had so far in this text by examining the various advantages and disadvantages associated with peer support work within mental health discourse today.

Notes

1 CHIME – Connectiveness, Hope, Identity, Meaning and Purpose, Empowerment – Leamy et al. (2011).
2 A tier 4 service is an intensive support team. They are essentially wards and intensive home treatment.
3 Child and Adolescent Mental Health Services.

References

Abraham, K.M., Erickson, P., Sata, M.J. & Lewis, S.B. (2021) Job satisfaction and burnout among peer support specialists: The contribution of supervisory mentorship, recovery-oriented workplaces and role clarity. *Advances in Mental Health* 20(1), 1–13. https://doi.org/10.1080/18387357.2021.1977667

Adams, W.E., Duquette, R., de Wet, A. & Rogers, E.S. (2023) Competing allegiance in an unclear role: Peer and non-peer understanding of peer support in Massachusetts, United States. *SSM-Mental Health* 4, 100245. https://doi.org/10.1016/j.ssmmh.2023.100245

Anthony, W.A. (1993) Recovery from mental illness: The guiding vision of the mental health service system in the 1990s. *Psychosocial Rehabilitation Journal* 16(4), 11–23. https://doi.org/10.1037/h0095655

Archard, P.J., O'Reilly, M., Spilsbury, T., Ali, A., Kulik, L. & Solanki, P. (2023) Informality, advocacy and the sharing of lived experiences in peer support work. *Irish Journal of Psychological Medicine* https://doi.org/10.1017/ipm.2023.8

Atlantic Technological University (2022) *Certificate in Peer Support Practice* (Internet) Available at: www.gmit.ie/certificate-in-peer-support-practice (Accessed 17 November 2024).

Bailie, A.H. (2015) *"From the Same Mad Planet" A Grounded Theory Study of Service User Accounts of the Relationship that Develops within Professional Peer Support Work* (Published PhD Dissertation). University of Nottingham, United Kingdom.

Barlow, C.A., Schiff, J.W., Chugh, U., Rawlinson, D., Hides, E. & Leith, J. (2010) An evaluation of a suicide bereavement peer support program. *Death Studies* 34(10), 915–930. https://doi.org/10.1080/07481181003761435

Barr, K.R., Townsend, M.L. & Grenyer, B.F.S. (2020) Using peer workers with lived experience to support the treatment of borderline personality disorder: A qualitative study of consumer, carer and clinician perspectives. *Borderline Personality Disorder and Emotional Disregulation* 7, 20. https://doi.org/10.1186/s40479-020-00135-5

Berry, C., Hayward, M.I. & Chandler, R. (2011) Another rather than other: Experiences of peer support specialist workers and their managers working in mental health services. *Journal of Public Mental Health* 10(4), 238–249. https://doi.org/10.1108/17465721111188269

Cabral, L., Strother, H., Muhr, K., Sefton, L. & Savageau, J. (2014) Clarifying the role of the mental health peer specialist in Massachusetts, USA: Insights from peer specialists, supervisors and clients. *Health and Social Care in the Community* 22(1), 104–112. https://doi.org/10.1111/hsc.12072

Cha, B.S., Borghouts, J., Eikey, E., Mukamel, D.B., Schueller, S.M., Sorkin, D.H., Stadnick, N.A., Zhao, X., Zheng, K. & Schneider, M.L. (2024) Variability in the integration of peers in a multi-site digital mental health innovation project. *Administration and Policy in Mental Health and Mental Health Services Research* 51, 226–239. https://doi.org/10.1007/s10488-023-01331-5

Chikezie, C. (2024) Lived experience of direct provision. In *Peer Support Work: Practice, Training and Implementation* (Mahon, D. ed.). Emerald Publishing Limited, Leeds, pp. 61–71.

Copeland, M.E. (2018) *Wellness Recovery Action Plan.* Human Potential Press, Sudbury, Massachusetts.

Davidson, L., Chinman, M., Sells, D. & Rowe, M. (2006) Peer support among adults with serious mental illness: A report from the field. *Schizophrenia Bulletin* 32, 443–450. https://doi.org/10.1093/schbul/sbj043

Erondu, C. & McGraw, C. (2021) Exploring the barriers and enablers to the implementation and adoption of recovery orientated practice by community mental health provider organisations in England. *Social Work in Mental Health* 19(5), 457–475. https://doi.org/10.1080/15332985.2021.1949426

Faulkner, A., Sadd, J., Hughes, A., Thompson, S., Nettle, M., Wallcraft, J., Collar, J., de la Huye, S. & McKinley, S. (2013) *Mental Health Peer Support in England: Piecing Together the Jigsaw* (Internet). Available at: www.mind.org.uk/media-a/4096/piecing-together-the-jigsaw-full-version.pdf (Accessed 2 November 2024).

Gillard, S., Banach, N., Barlow, E., Byrne, J., Foster, R., Goldsmith, L., Marks, J., McWilliam, C., Morshead, R., Stepanian, K., Turner, R., Verey, A. & White, S. (2021) Developing and testing a principle-based fidelity index for peer support in mental health services. *Social Psychiatry and Psychiatric Epidemiology* 56, 1903–1911. https://doi.org/10.1007/s00127-021-02038-4

Gillard, S., Foster, R., Gibson, S., Goldsmith, L., Marks, J. & White, S. (2017) Describing a principles-based approach to developing and evaluating peer worker roles as peer support moves into mainstream mental health services. *Mental Health and Social Inclusion* 21(3), 133–143. https://doi.org/10.1108/MHSI-03-2017-0016

Gillard, S., Gibson, S.L., Holley, J. & Lucock, M. (2014) Developing a change model for peer worker interventions in mental health services: A qualitative research study. *Epidemiology and Psychiatric Sciences* 24(5), 435–445. https://doi.org/10.1017/S2045796014000407

Glynn, C. (2023) *The Battle of the Peer* (Internet). Available at: https://madinireland.com/2023/05/the-battle-of-the-peer/ (Accessed 28 October 2024).

Gray, B. & Sisto, M. (2024) Peer support work in hospital: A first person and lived experience guide. *Schizophrenia Bulletin Open* 5(1), sgad035. https://doi.org/10.1093/schizbullopen/sgad035

Harty, M. (2024) Peer support work within the traveller community. In *Peer Support Work: Practice, Training and Implementation* (Mahon, D. ed.). Emerald Publishing, Leeds, pp. 83–94.

Health Service Executive (n.d.) *Toolkit to Support Peer Support Workers Working in the Health Service Executive* (Internet). Available at: www.hse.ie/eng/services/list/4/mental-health-services/mentalhealthengagement/peer-support-workers-toolkit.pdf (Accessed 3 November 2024).

Health Service Executive (2020) *Peer Support Distance Working: Guidance on A Model of Peer Support Working during the Covid-19 Pandemic* (Internet). Available at: www.hse.ie/eng/services/list/4/mental-health-services/mental-health-engagement-and-recovery/peer-support-distance-working.pdf (Accessed 3 November 2024).

Heon, T. (2024) *The Integration of Peer Support Principles in Community Mental Health Policy and Practice: Towards Epistemic Humility* (Internet). Available at: www.madinamerica.com/2024/02/integration-peer-support/ (Accessed 1 December 2024).

Honey, A., Hancock, N., Barton, R., Berry, B., Gilroy, J., Glover, H., Hines, M., Waks, S. & Wells, K. (2023) How do mental health services foster hope? Experience of people accessing services. *Community Mental Health Journal* 59(5), 894–903. https://doi.org/10.1007/s10597-022-01073-y

Hunt, E. & Byrne, M. (2019) *Peer Support Workers in Mental Health Services: A report on the Impact of Peer Support Workers in Mental Health Services* (Internet). Available at: www.lenus.ie/bitstream/handle/10147/635104/peer-support-workers-in-mental-health-services.pdf?sequence=1&isAllowed=y (Accessed 2 November 2024).

Intentional Peer Support (2024) *About* (Internet). Available at: www.intentionalpeersupport.org/about/?v=b8a74b2fbcbb#:~:text=Shery%20M ead%2C%20Founder,house%20and%20a%20limited%20future (Accessed 28 October 2024).

Janouskova, M., Vickova, K., Harcuba, V., Kluckova, T., Motlova, J. & Motlova, L.B. (2022) The challenges of inter-role conflict for peer support workers. *Psychiatric Services* 72(12), 1424–1427. https://doi.org/10.1176/appi.ps.202100566

Jacobson, N., Trojanowski, L. & Dewa, C.S. (2012) What do peer support workers do? A job description. *BMC Health Services Research* 12, 205. https://doi.org/10.1186/1472-6963-12-205

Johnsen, T.L., Eriksen, H.R., Indahl, A. & Tveito, T.H. (2017) Directive and nondirective social support in the workplace – Is this social support distinction important for subjective health complaints, job satisfaction, and perception of job demands and job control? *Scandinavian Journal of Public Health* 46(3), 358–367. https://doi.org/10.1177/1403494817726617

Kemp, V. & Henderson, A.R. (2012) Challenges faced by mental health peer support workers: Peer support from the peer supporter's point of view. *Psychiatric Rehabilitation Journal* 35(4), 337–340. http://dx.doi.org/10.2975/35.4.2012.337.340

Kirkegaard, S. & Andersen, D. (2022) Peer workers as emotion managers: Tight and loose enactment of mutuality in mental health care. *SSM – Qualitative Research in Health* 2, 100200. https://doi.org/10.1016/j.ssmqr.2022.100200

Krumm, S., Haun, M., Hiller, S., Charles, A., Kalha, J., Niwemuhwezi, J., Nixdorf, R., Puschner, B., Ryan, G., Shamba, D., Epstein, P.G. & Moran, G. (2022) Mental health worker's perspectives on peer support in high-, middle- and low income settings: A focus group study. *BMC Psychiatry* 22, 604. https://doi.org/10.1186/s12888-022-04206-5

Kumar, A., Azevedo, K.J., Factor, A., Hailu, E., Ramirez, J., Lindley, S.E. & Jain, S. (2019) Peer support in an outpatient program for veterans with posttraumatic stress disorder: Translating participants experiences into a recovery model. *Psychological Services* 16(3), 415–424. https://doi.org/10.1037/ser0000269

Leamy, M., Bird, V., Le Boutillier, C., Williams, J. & Slade, M. (2011) Conceptual frame-work for personal recovery in mental health: Systematic review and narrative synthesis. *British Journal of Psychiatry* 199(6), 445–452. https://doi.org/10.1192/bjp.bp.110.083733

Lernnox, R., Lamarche, L. & O'Shea, T. (2021) Peer support workers as a bridge: A qualita-tive study exploring the role of peer support workers in the care of people who use drugs during and after hospitalization. *Harm Reduction Journal* 18, 19. https://doi.org/10.1186/s12954-021-00467-7

Mahon, D. (2023) A systematic scoping review of interventions delivered by peers to sup-port the resettlement of refugees and asylum seekers. *Mental Health and Social Inclusion* 26(1). https://doi.org/10.1108/MHSI-12-2021-0085

Mayer, C. & McKenzie, K. (2017) "….it shows that there's no limit": The psychological impact of co-production for experts by experience working in youth mental health. *Health and Social Care in the Community* 25(3), 1181–1189. https://doi.org/10.1111/hsc.12418

Mead, S. (2014) *Intentional Peer Support: An Alternative Approach.* Intentional Peer Support, West Chesterfield.

Mead, S. (2019) *Intentional Peer Support Core Material 2019.* Intentional Peer Support, West Chesterfield.

Moll, S., Holmes, J., Geronimo, J. & Sherman, D. (2009) Work transitions for peer support providers in traditional mental health programs: Unique challenges and opportunities. *Work* 33, 449–458. https://doi.org/10.3233/WOR-2009-0893

Mullineaux, L.M. (2017) *Service User Experiences of Peer Support in an Adult Community Mental Health Service: An Interpretative Phenomenological Analysis.* Doctorate Dissertation, Published, University of East Anglia, United Kingdom.

Naughton, L., Collins, P. & Ryan, M. (2015) *Peer Support Workers – A Guidance Paper* (Internet). Available at: www.lenus.ie/bitstream/handle/10147/576059/PeerSupportW orkersAGuidance Paper.pdf?sequence=6&isAllowed=y (Accessed 28 October 2024).

Nguyen, J., Goldsmith, L., Rains, L.S. & Gillard, S. (2022) Peer support in early interven-tion in psychosis: A qualitative research study. *Journal of Mental Health* 31(2), 196–202. https://doi.org/10.1080/09638237.2021.1922647

NHS England (2023) *Supported Self-Management: Peer Support Guide* (Internet). Available at: www.england.nhs.uk/long-read/peer-support/ (Accessed 17 November 2024).

Norton, M.J. (2022) More than just a health care assistant: Peer support working within rehabilitation and recovery mental health services. *Irish Journal of Psychological Medicine*. https://doi.org/10.1017/ipm.2022.32

Norton, M.J. (2023) Peer support working: A question of ontology and epistemology. *International Journal of Mental Health Systems* 17, 1. https://doi.org/10.1186/s13033-023-00570-1

Norton, M.J. (2024a) Peer work in mental health services. In *Peer Support Work: Practice, Training and Implementation* (Mahon, D. ed.). Emerald Publishing, Leeds, pp. 9–23.

Norton, M.J. (2024b) Using learned tools for experiential gain: The application of experien-tial knowledge to traditional service processes. *Irish Journal of Psychological Medicine* 1–2. https://doi.org/10.1017/ipm.2024.4

Norton, M.J., Archard, P. & Swords, C. (2023) The ethics of informality and dual rela-tionships in peer support. *Psychiatric Services* 74(2), 2. https://doi.org/10.1176/appi.ps.20230291

Norton, M.J. & Cuskelly, K. (2021) Family recovery interventions with families of mental health service users: A systematic review of the literature. *International Journal of*

Environmental Research and Public Health 18(15), 7858. https://doi.org/10.3390/ijerph1 8157858

O'Donnell, C. & Cusack, A. (2024) Homelessness and peer work. In *Peer Support Work: Practice, Training and Implementation* (Mahon, D. ed.). Emerald Publishing, Leeds, pp. 43–57.

Panaite, A-C., Desroches, O-A., Warren, E., Rouly, G., Castonguay, G. & Boivin, A. (2024) Engaging with peers to integrate community care: Knowledge synthesis and conceptual map. *Health Expectations* 27(2), e14034. https://doi.org/10.1111/hex.14034

Pattoni, L. (2012) *Strengths-Based Approaches for Working with Individuals* (Internet). Available at: www.iriss.org.uk/resources/insights/strengths-based-approaches-working-individuals (Accessed 3 November 2024).

Paulson, R., Herinckx, H., Demmler, J., Clarke, G., Cutler, D. & Birecree, E. (1999) Comparing practice patterns of consumers and non-consumer mental health service providers. *Community Mental Health Journal* 35(3), 251–269. https://doi.org/10.1023/A:1018745403590

Peer Advocacy in Mental Health (n.d.) *What Is Peer Advocacy in Mental Health* (Internet). Available at: www.peeradvocacyinmentalhealth.com/mission#:~:text=Peer%20Advocacy%20in%20Mental%20Health%20is…&text=Providing%20and%20discussing%20options.,decision%2Dmaking%20by%20the%20individual.&text=Promoting%20self%2Dadvocacy%20through%20empowerment,in%20their%20treatment%20and%20care (Accessed 17 November 2024).

Price,V. (2021) *Hope: A Personal Reflection about the Role of Hope in Peer Support* (Internet). Available at: www.peerhub.co.uk/post/hope-a-personal-reflection-about-the-role-of-hope-in-peer-support (Accessed 3 November 2024).

Rapp, C.A. & Sullivan, W.P. (2014) The strenghts model: Birth to toddlerhood. *Advances in Social Work* 15(1), 129–142. https://doi.org/10.18060/16643

Reeves, V., McIntyre, H., Loughhjead, M., Halpin, M.A. & Procter, N. (2024) Actions targeting the integration of peer workforce in mental health organisations: A mixed-methods systematic review. *BMC Psychiatry* 24, 211. https://doi.org/10.1186/s12888-024-05664-9

Repper, J., Aldridge, B., Gilfoyle, S., Gillard, S., Perkins, R. & Rennison, J. (2013) *Peer Support Workers: Theory and Practice* (Internet) Available at: https://static1.squaresp ace.com/static/65e873c27971d37984653be0/t/668ce21ba54f933596890e57/172050 8956537/5ImROC-Peer-Support-Workers-Theory-and-Practice.pdf   (Accessed   2 November 2024).

Rosenburg, D. & Argentzell, E. (2018) Service users experiences of peer support in Swedish mental health care: A "tipping point" in the care-giving culture. *Journal of Psychosocial Rehabilitation and Mental Health* 5, 53–61. https://doi.org/10.1007/s40737-018-0109-1

SAMHSA (n.d.) *Core Competencies for Peer Workers* (Internet). Available at: www.samhsa. gov/technical-assistance/brss-tacs/peer-support-workers/core-competencies (Accessed 2 November 2024).

SAMHSA (2015) *Core Competencies for Peer Workers in Behavioural Health Services* (Internet). Available at: www.samhsa.gov/sites/default/files/programs_campaigns/brss_t acs/core-competencies_508_12_13_18.pdf (Accessed 2 November 2024).

Schiavon, C.C., Marchetti, E., Gurgel, L.G., Busnello, F.M. & Reppold, C.T. (2017) Optimism and hope in chronic disease: A systematic review. *Frontiers in Psychology* 7, 2022. https://doi.org/10.3389/fpsyg.2016.02022

Schrank, B., Hayward, M., Stanghellini, G. & Davidson, L. (2011) Hope in psychiatry. *Advances in Psychiatric Treatment* 17, 227–235. https://doi.org/10.1192/apt.bp.109.007286

Skills for Health (n.d.) *Peer Support Roles in the Mental Health Workforce – Examples of Current Practice: Recognising the Benefit of 'Lived' Experience* (Internet). Available at: www.skillsforhealth.org.uk/images/resource-section/service-area/personalisation/peer-support-report09-2011.pdf (Accessed 1 December 2024).

South Eastern Health and Social Care Trust (n.d.) Peer Advocacy (Internet). Available at: https://setrust.hscni.net/service/peer-advocacy/#:~:text=Peer%20Advocates%20will%20support%20people,a%20group%20 0with%20similar%20issues (Accessed 17 November 2024).

Stefancic, A., Bochicchio, L., Tuda, D., Harris, Y., DeSomma, K. & Cabassa, L.J. (2021) Strategies and lessons learned for supporting and supervising peer specialists. *Psychiatric Services* 72, 606–609. https://doi.org/10.1176/appi.ps.202000515

The Housing Agency (n.d.) *Peer Support Specialist Toolkit: Integration and Delivery of Peer Support Specialist Services* (Internet). Available at: www.housingagency.ie/sites/default/files/2024- 09/The%20Housing%20Agency%20103982_Peer%20Support%20Specialist%20Tool kit_FINAL.pdf (Accessed 1 December 2024).

The Workplace Mediation (2023) *The Role of Peer Support Progams in Conflict Resolution* (Internet) Available at: https://theworkplacemediator.co.uk/the-role-of-peer-support-programs-in-conflict-resolution/ (Accessed 1 December 2024).

Thiele, L., Zorn, V. & Kauffeld, S. (2019) Quid pro quo? The benefit of reciprocity, multiplexity, and multireciprocity in early career peer support. *Applied Network Science* 4, 7. https://doi.org/10.1007/s41109-019-0118-3

Usideme, O.I. (2024) Peer support in ethnic minorities communities. In *Peer Support Work: Practice, Training and Implementation* (Mahon, D. ed.). Emerald Publishing, Leeds, pp. 73–82.

Viking, T., Wenzer, J., Hylin, U. & Nilsson, L. (2022) Peer support workers' role and expertise and interprofessional learning in mental health care: A scoping review. *Journal of Interprofessional Care* 36(6), 828–838. https://doi.org/10.1080/13561820.2021.2014796

Vocabulary.com (2024) *Principle* (Internet). Available at: www.vocabulary.com/dictionary/principle#:~:text=A%20principle%20is%20a %20kind,guide)%20most%20people%20and%20businesses (Accessed 2 November 2024).

Walde, P., Hadala, J., Peipe, V. & Vollm, B.A. (2023) Implementation of a peer support worker in a forensic psychiatric hospital in Germany – Views of patients. *Frontiers in Psychiatry* 8(14), 1061106. https://doi.org/10.3389/fpsyt.2023.1061106

Watson, E. (2019) What is peer support? History, evidence and values. In *Peer Support in Mental Health* (Watson, E. & Meddings, S. eds.). Red Globe Press, London, pp. 6–24.

Wright, M. & Mahon, D. (2024) Addiction and peer support work. In *Peer Support Work: Practice, Training and Implementation* (Mahon, D. ed.). Emerald Publishing, Leeds, pp. 25–34.

Xie, H. (2013) Strengths-based approach for mental health recovery. *Iranian Journal of Psychiatry and Behavioural Sciences* 7(2), 5–10.

Appendix: Sample Peer Support Worker Job Specification

Job Title and Grade	Peer Support Worker (Grade Code)
Campaign Reference	
Closing Date	
Proposed Interview Date	
Location of Post	
Informal Enquiries	
Details of Service	
Reporting Relationship	The post holder will report directly to the nominated line manager.
Purpose of the Post	The Peer Support Worker will be a full and integral member of the multi-disciplinary team, providing formalised peer support and practical assistance to people using our services and their supporters (families/carers) in helping them regain control over their lives and their own unique Recovery Journey. The Peer Support Worker will use their expertise gained through lived experience to inspire hope and recovery as per xxxx. They will facilitate and support information sharing to promote choice, self-determination and opportunities for connection with local communities and may link with other developments through a range of integrated and community-based support programmes. As a member of the multi-disciplinary team, the Peer Support Worker will work alongside people using our services on a one-to-one and/or group basis. They will work under the supervision of line management. The Peer Support Worker will take an active role in promoting recovery values within the service in which they work, and act as a champion for Recovery for xxx with external agencies and organisations.
Principal Duties and Responsibilities	*Under the direction of the nominated line manager the Peer Support Worker will:* **Professional/Admin** • Work as a member of the multi-disciplinary team to deliver support to people using our services and where appropriate their supporters. (family members/carers) (Assist people using our services to identify their needs, strengths, personal interests, and goals.) • Manage a caseload with the Community Mental Health Team (CMHT) in line with caseload review practices.

Job Title and Grade	Peer Support Worker (Grade Code)
	• Contribute, as appropriate, from a recovery perspective to the assessment, planning, implementation and review of individual care plans with the multi-disciplinary team. • Maintain all written records as per Health Service Executive (HSE) policies. • Have a working knowledge of xxxx standards as they apply to the role. • Maintain professional standards with regard to service user and data confidentiality. • Demonstrate pro-active commitment to all communications with internal and external stakeholders • Keep up-to-date with organisational developments within xxx. • Work in accordance with the principles and values of recovery as described in xxxx. **Customer Service/ Service Delivery** • Ensure that service users are treated with dignity and respect. • Support the person using our services and be aware of their rights within the service and the supports available to access these. • Be aware of the Human Rights legislation in relation to the requirements of this post. • Promote equality of opportunity and good relations as outlined in xxxx Policy • Facilitate opportunities for people using our services to direct their own recovery, based on recovery principles. • Promote and support independent living for people using our services, signposting to their local community and developing connections with family, friends and significant others where appropriate. • Through discussion and consultation with the service user, identify solutions, set goals, plan and move through and beyond the service as part of the individual care planning process. This process will be achieved by using a recovery process. • Act on feedback from service users / customers and report same to Line Manager. **Health and Safety** • Promote a safe working environment in accordance with xxx legislation. • Be aware of and implement agreed policies, procedures and safe professional practice by adhering to relevant legislation, regulations and standards.

(Continued)

Job Title and Grade	Peer Support Worker (Grade Code)
	• Actively participate in risk management issues, identify risks and take responsibility for appropriate action. • Document appropriately and report any adverse incidents, near misses, hazards and accidents in accordance with organisational guidelines. • Have a working knowledge of the xxx standards as they apply to the role, for example xxx. • Support, promote and actively participate in sustainable energy, water and waste initiatives to create a more sustainable, low-carbon and efficient health service. **Education and Training** • Attend induction and mandatory in-service education relevant to the role. • Participate in the induction of new staff as directed. • Participate in Performance Achievement in conjunction with the line manager. • Participate in team-based development, education, training and learning

Essential Eligibility Criteria Qualifications and/or Experience	**Candidates must have by the closing date for receipt of applications for this post:**
	
	1. Professional Qualifications, Experience etc.
	  b. Hold accreditation, at the appropriate grade and standard in peer support work in mental health.
	  And
	c. Have experience working (paid or voluntary) with individuals with mental health needs
	2. Health
	  A candidate for and any person holding the office must be fully competent and capable of undertaking the duties attached to the office and be in a state of health such as would indicate a reasonable prospect of ability to render regular and efficient service.
	3. Character
	  Each candidate for and any person holding the office must be of good character.

Other Requirements	• Have personal lived experience of mental health difficulties including insight into the recovery process. • Access to appropriate personal transport is a necessary requirement to carry out the duties and responsibilities of this post. • Ability to work in a flexible way, which may include evenings, weekends, bank and public holidays.

Job Title and Grade	Peer Support Worker (Grade Code)
Skills, Competencies and/or Knowledge	*Candidates must demonstrate the following:* **Professional Knowledge:** • Insight and understanding of the personal recovery process and what that may involve for individual people using our services and using the individual peer support worker's recovery story to support others. • Knowledge and experience of self-care frameworks and approaches in the context of mental health recovery. • Knowledge of the basic structure of the CMHT and HSE Mental Health Services. • Knowledge of the xxx policy. • Knowledge and understanding of the importance of self-care and associated techniques, from a recovery perspective. • Experience in delivering a variety of group activities that support and strengthen recovery. Have examples of tools/methods used in mental health recovery and social inclusion. • Basic knowledge of Information and Communication Technology (ICT). **Planning and Organising Skills** • Organisational and time management skills to meet objectives within agreed timeframes and achieve quality results • The ability to work to tight deadlines and operate effectively with multiple competing priorities. **Evaluating Information and Decision-Making** • The ability to assess complex information from a variety of sources and make effective decisions. • Effective problem-solving and decision-making skills. **Leadership and Teamwork** • Teamwork skills including the ability to work in a multi-disciplinary team environment (i.e. in a team with other disciplines). • The capacity to operate successfully in a challenging operational environment while adhering to quality standards. • Motivation and an innovative approach to the job within a changing working environment. • The ability to work independently, in a range of settings and as appropriate.

(Continued)

Job Title and Grade	Peer Support Worker (Grade Code)
	Commitment to Providing a Quality Service • A service user focuses on the delivery of services. • A core belief in and passion for the sustainable delivery of high-quality service user-focused services. • Commitment to recovery-focused principles and practices. • Commitment to continuing professional development. **Communication and Interpersonal Skills** • Effective interpersonal skills. • Effective written and verbal communication skills; including the ability to present information in a clear and concise manner. • The ability to form peer relationships with people using our services and supportive relationships with family members. • The ability to interact in a professional manner with other Mental Health staff and other key stakeholders.
Campaign-Specific Selection Process Ranking/Shortlisting/ Interview	
Code of Practice	

Chapter 5

Advantages of and Challenges to Peer Support Work

Case Study Contributor:

Nicole Troy

5.1 Introduction

As we now know, introducing a new role into existing multi-disciplinary team structures to compliment traditional care pathways is a complex process, requiring much work on both the developmental and evaluation stages of role integration (O'Dwyer, 2018). To date, there has been considerable work conducted on this, both in Ireland and internationally (Norton et al., 2023). These processes have occurred in a slow and patchy manner, but ultimately, they led to the professionalisation of peer support services within mental health service provision (Chinman et al., 2014; Gordon and Bradstreet, 2015; Adams, 2020). These, along with other macro, meso and micro factors, have led to a number of advantages and challenges to peer support work within a mental health realm which needs further exploration and synthesis (Glynn, 2023; Saad et al., 2024).

This chapter explores these advantages and challenges from a micro to macro perspective. In Section 5.2 the advantages of peer support work within mental health service provision are explored. This is an essential element of the chapter as, in essence, it is providing the rationale as to why peers should be involved in the treatment of other service users within mental health services. Section 5.3 discusses the barriers and challenges to peer support work from a mental health context. It also lays the foundations for some of the topics we will discuss later in this book, for example Chapter 8. Section 5.4 concludes with a summary of this chapter and how this has improved our understanding of peer support work in mental health which we can use to understand other key concepts explored in this text. It will also refer to the following chapter of this text.

5.2 Advantages of Peer Support Work within Mental Health Service Provision

Since the integration of peer support, the concept has brought about a number of advantages. Solomon (2004) showed, in their paper, a number of benefits, which has also been noted by numerous other authors, both nationally and internationally. Such advantages have been documented in a variety of publications ranging in quality from academic, peer reviewed journals to college theses as well as the grey

DOI: 10.4324/9781032717050-7

literature. In this particular analysis of these various sources of text, the advantages of peer support work could be documented at two levels moving from the micro (individual/Peer Support Worker) to the macro (service/organisation) level. Such advantages are discussed in the following section.

5.2.1 Advantages of the Individual Service User

There is a growing amount of literature that demonstrates the efficacy or benefit of peer support work at an individual, service user level (Faulkner and Basset, 2010). Indeed, the benefits of peer support work for the service user can be aligned to the CHIME framework,[1] which contains the concepts necessary for personal recovery to occur (Leamy et al., 2011).

The first concept within CHIME is connectiveness. Within the peer support work literature, Mullineaux (2017) begins this discussion by highlighting that one of the most positive/beneficial aspects of peer support work is the personal narrative – with particular attention to the sharing of the same. As we will later reveal, there are debates within the literature about how lived experience, brought to life through personal narratives, should be shared. For more information on this debate, see Chapter 6. Regardless of how the personal narrative is shared, it is said to have a cathartic effect on both individuals, thereby allowing service users – in this case, the recipients of the narrative – to feel less alone in terms of their suffering (Mullineaux, 2017) and more connected to the peer they are working with. Sells et al. (2008) add to Mullineaux's work by suggesting that the sharing of narratives creates a type of mutuality and connection, whereby the mere presence of the Peer Support Worker alone becomes enough to create a positive effect on the service user's mental health and well-being. This close relationship, as discussed in a later chapter,[2] also positively impacts service utilisation as individual service users who are under the care of a Peer Support Worker are 64% more likely to seek help for their mental health difficulties as a result of direct peer involvement in their care (Cheesmond et al., 2020).

Second, the concept associated with CHIME is hope. Bouchard et al. (2010) identified that Peer Support Workers increase a person's sense of hope for the future. This may occur due to the peer's role modelling function[3] (The Housing Agency, 2024). However, it can also be achieved through the peer's relationship with the connectiveness-based benefits. These benefits all support the deflation of feelings of loneliness associated with a burden of experiencing mental health difficulties (Beeble and Salem, 2009).

Third, the concept within the CHIME framework is identity. Here, Peer Support Workers, in the work they do with service users, can support these same individuals to see themselves beyond the passive service user/patient identity to a new identity – often that of a role model to other service users within the services who may be at the beginning of their self-defined personal recovery journey (Davidson et al., 1999). In terms of identity, this change begins from the start of the peer relationship with service users as the relationship lacks professionalism. This lack of professionalism makes the relationship so informal that it resembles a friend-like partnership, which is important and necessary for the relationship to be therapeutic (Meehan et al., 2002).[4] This, as we will explore in later chapters, occurs because the role of Peer Support Worker is observed by service users as informal in nature, thereby creating a space where hierarchical structures often present within other professional relationships is essentially removed allowing for the creation of a semi-buddy relationship – a state known as informality (Moll et al., 2009; Norton, 2022). Within this state of informality, labels are eradicated and as such, the individual is seen as a person as opposed to their diagnostic label.

All these then link to CHIME's fourth element: meaning and purpose, as resulting from the above activities, a person's recovery journey from mental health challenges is positively influenced (Cabral et al., 2014; Hunt and Byrne, 2019). Such areas positively impacted an individual's well-being, self-esteem and social skills (Gray and Sisto, 2024). This finding was also noted by Boardman et al. (2014), who identified a causal link between peer support interventions and the service user's overall mental state. Bouchard et al. (2010) add to this by suggesting that such elements of a person's mental state positively impacted by peer support include the service user's behaviour and emotions leading to improved conduct and communication pathways between stakeholders. In this way, Peer Support Workers can act as buffers among stakeholders (Smedberg, 2015). Cooper et al. (2024) say that Peer Support Workers can be uncovered through the process of an umbrella review of the available literature as peer support can be effective in improving certain clinical outcomes, including self-efficacy and recovery. Finally, peer support has also been shown to have a positive impact on a service user's global functioning scores[5] both at six-month and yearly intervals, thereby enhancing the functional aspect of their personal recovery journey (Roelandt et al., 2024).

The final element of the CHIME framework is that of empowerment. Like the four previous elements, peer support work also has the effect of empowering individuals along their personal recovery journey. Through the peer's ability to work through the system, individual service users can gain access to educational resources that empower them to move forward in their recovery journey so that they can become active members of their social world and indeed society at large (Repper et al., 2013). Such educational resources do this by allowing the individual to make sense of their current life situation, thereby allowing the service user to reflect and make positive changes towards their personal recovery journey (Bouchard et al., 2010). Finally, such resources can lead to the development of social skills and the creation of new networks (Walker and Bryant, 2013). All these are useful to support service users to become once again actively involved in their communities (Hunt and Byrne, 2019).

5.2.2 Advantageous to the Peer Support Worker

Interestingly, as a Peer Support Worker, providing support to those in an earlier phase of recovery has a reciprocal effect that impacts not just the service user in receipt of peer support but also the Peer Support Worker themselves (Boardman et al., 2015; Naughton et al., 2015; Smedberg, 2015; Kim and Kweon, 2024). In fact, quantitative evidence from Bracke et al. (2008) suggests that providing peer support is more beneficial than receiving it. However, in this section, we will not compare the advantages for the service user to that of the peer. Instead, this section and indeed this chapter have been constructed to demonstrate the evidence currently available into peer support work in mental health based on their benefits and challenges.

Firstly, being employed as a Peer Support Worker has been proven to empower the peer in their life-long recovery journey (Salzer and Shear, 2002). Faulkner and Basset (2010) add to this by suggesting that such empowerment comes from putting the peer's lived experience of mental distress to good use. As noted by Austin et al. (2014), other benefits come from supporting others on their recovery journey and include increased positive self-identity, identification of a sense of achievement and positivity. Mowbray et al. (1998) add to the above by suggesting that being employed as a peer worker has a number of benefits, including improvements in the individual's economic situation, increased sense of self-worth, as well as increased ability to be assertive within relationships. Additionally, simply enacting peer support work was shown to benefit the peer worker by improving their overall mental health and well-being, reducing the frequency of usage of services, increasing their functionality and skills development in gaining a renewed sense of purpose in one's life (Bouchard et al., 2010; Burke et al., 2018).

On peer's enacted role, Chang et al. (2016) found that Peer Support Workers generally have higher job satisfaction rates compared to their non-peer colleagues. Similarly from an organisational perspective, the wage a peer receives for their work seems sufficient enough for these peers to live on according to Smith (2024). However, this is not reflected in the feedback from peers as they have experienced little satisfaction when it came to monetary gain and job progression/promotion opportunities (Chang et al., 2016).

5.2.3 Advantages of the Services/Organisation

Not only the user and provider of the service have peer support work advantages, but also they have some macro, organisational advantages. Within services, the presence of the Peer Support Worker is essential for these said services to achieve the aspirations identified in policy (Byrne et al., 2017a). As noted in Chapter 10, the aspirations of policy currently are towards user involvement and recovery (Department of Health, 2020; Health Service Executive, 2024). Peers are believed to support services in this endeavour as they provide a unique perspective on service-related issues due to their lived experience of mental health difficulties, lived understanding of recovery, as well as its related values and concepts (Byrne et al., 2015). Ehrlich et al. (2020) add to Byrne and colleagues' point suggesting that peers also are able to carry out this function as they are the catalysts for the conduction of frank conversations that allows for changes in practices to occur in traditional staff towards recovery orientation. As such, they support non-peer staff to see the possibilities of recovery (Smedberg, 2015).

Peer Support Workers also have an essential impact on an MDT level. Within MDTs, peers have a role in eliminating negative attitudes towards the individuals the personnel that make up the MDT work with. This is beneficial as it allows traditional staff to release any residual hierarchical power associated with their role, so that they can more authentically support service users in their care (Repper et al., 2013; Blash et al., 2015). Additionally, it allows these staff members to be less stigmatising towards those they support (Gillard et al., 2014). For the service user, the presence of the peer on MDTs supports these individuals in trusting the system with their mental well-being and recovery journey (Dixon et al., 1994; Bennetts et al., 2011; Walker and Bryant, 2013; Blash et al., 2015; Rosenberg and Argentzell, 2018). Byrne et al. (2016) expand on this finding, suggesting that the peer's presence alone is enough to facilitate the construction of a recovery environment within a backdrop of a biomedically led culture. The effects of this are noted by Repper et al. (2013) as the elimination of discriminating language and medical jargon used by non-peer, traditional staff over the course of their work.

In addition to the transformation of the traditional culture based on the presence of the peer, they also have a benefit at an organisational level through the economic savings associated with the role. Both Min et al. (2007) and Sledge et al. (2011) have identified a significant reduction in re-hospitalisation rates that can be directly attributed to the activity of Peer Support Workers. In those that are re-hospitalised, Peer Support Workers were also linked to a significant reduction in the number of bed days[6] spent within psychiatric hospitals (Sledge et al., 2011; Trachtenberg et al., 2013; Austin et al., 2014). An example presented by Trachtenberg and colleagues suggests that for every £1 spent on Peer Support Workers, services save on average £2 on psychiatric hospital beds. However, the evidence regarding these claims should be taken with the knowledge that overall the evidence relating to these claims remains inconsistent with Clarke et al's (2000) findings contradicting those presented above.

5.3 Challenges to Peer Support Work within Mental Health Service Provision

Like the advantages listed above, the literature examined also identified a number of challenges to peer support work. The challenges explored here yet again come from a micro (service user/Peer Support Worker) level to a macro (system/organisational) level. As noted below, most of the challenges centre on the role of the Peer Support Worker or how the role is implemented and accepted within the wider system (Hunt and Byrne, 2019; Griffin, 2022). These challenges are now explored, beginning with challenges from the individual service user discussed in Section 5.3.1.

5.3.1 Challenges from Individual Service User

As demonstrated here, when it comes to the challenges to peer support work, little to no evidence of challenges comes from the service user population. The exception to this is from both Bouchard et al. (2010) and Boardman et al. (2015), who suggest that service users themselves can become a potential barrier due to their withdrawn attitudes. However, Boardman and colleagues in particular note that this may have been caused by the severity of the mental health challenge and/or the treatment regimens used to treat the underlying psychopathology.

5.3.2 Challenges from the Peer Support Worker

A number of challenges relay back to the role of the Peer Support Worker themselves. The first major challenge identified in the available literature is the peer's employment into the role of Peer Support Worker themselves. This, as noted by Byrne et al. (2017b), represents a huge risk for the person's recovery, as to carry out the role, one must essentially '*come out*' and expose oneself as a service user/ former service user of the mental health services. Additionally, this risk is further enflamed by the lack of occupational support for peers in their role (Robertson et al., 2024).

Once the peer enters the system, two major challenges arise: that of role clarity and the working relationship between the service user, the peer and the system they conduct this work in and for (Dixon et al., 1994; Berry et al., 2011; Miyamoto and Sono, 2012). The lack of role clarity stems from a number of factors including, but not limited to, the use of a generic job description rather than identifying specific duties that constitute a peer's role within the health system (Dixon et al., 1994; Smedberg, 2015). As a result, this can lead to issues where non-peer providers feel that their role is being encroached on, for example the peer supporting the service user in decision-making regarding medications – all of which can lead to further ostrication of the peer role by non-peer staff (Tsai, 2002; Meehan et al., 2002). However, as we will reveal in a later chapter,[7] peers may utilise similar techniques in the process of their work with service user to that of non-peer staff, but what makes this peer work actual is the knowledge set in which such tools and techniques are being expressed in a different way from that of the non-peer, thereby transforming the tool/technique into something that peers can use and make a positive impact (Norton, 2024b).

In addition, another documented challenge to the peer is time constraints (Boardman et al., 2015). In this study, Boardman and colleagues have imposed a time limit of 20 minutes per visit once a week to meet with service users and support them on aspects of their recovery journey. This, as Boardman later admits, is inefficient for the therapeutic work of peer support to occur. This is further explored by both Byrne et al. (2015) and Mullineaux (2017), in which they link this time constraint to the non-peer provider, where the provider is expected to see a set number of service users within a particular time period. However, Mullineaux (2017) suggests that if such time pressures are communicated to the service user, this would mitigate this challenge. This is an example where non-peer providers lack a basic understanding of peer support work in the recovery journey of service users.

Time also arose as a direct challenge to the Peer Support Worker; however, this time it relates back to their working hours, with many practising on a part time, haphazard basis, which impacts the rate in which these peers can integrated into traditional MDT structures (Moll et al., 2009).

The final challenge expressed in the literature that comes from the Peer Support Worker is the dual space they occupy as both professional and friend.[8] This dual space has been identified by Barlow et al. (2010) and Faulkner and Bassett (2010) as a challenge to peer support work. This is because central to the peer role is the balancing act that happens between professional (Peer Support Worker) and friend (fellow service user) identities (Moll et al., 2009). This links with the peer's difficulty with boundaries within the role as noted by Davidson et al. (2006). Interestingly, a recent study identified that this occupation of a dual role has been the major factor in making the Peer Support Worker role successful today (Akerblom et al., 2023). In our next case study, Nicole notes many of the abovementioned challenges when she tries to navigate a dual role in her practice as a Peer Support Worker and as a Behavioural Therapist.

Case Study 4   A Day in the Life of a Peer Support Worker

Nicole Troy

This case study presents a day in the life of someone who works as both a Peer Support Worker and a Behavioural Therapist. Currently, I work as a Behavioural Therapist as my full-time profession, and I facilitate a weekly peer support group on Thursday evenings, after work. I am grateful to be involved in both of these roles with the aim to support individuals who go through various mental health challenges. The roles can sometime complement each other but more often than not; I'm in between balancing the compassionate lived-experience approach, with the more formal, evidence-based methods of my clinical work. Maintaining both roles can be multifaceted and complex, especially when flipping from various perspectives all in one day. Somehow, I can't help but get intertwined in both perspectives and adopting a strengths-based approach throughout both roles, as I sometime think, we are our own worst critiques and can often fail to find a good word or quality about ourselves. Within the peer support role, I've provided emotional support, shared lived experiences of various challenges and suggested various coping strategies that I have used for myself through darker times many years ago and now have the opportunity to share them, rather than what I was asked to implement by a professional. On a multitude of occasions, I've gained valuable knowledge from the peer support members and their experiences, which made me aware of how and why some of the health services in Ireland are continuing to let people down. This insight allows me to understand and acknowledge what is happening to individuals currently within the system and has also assessed my own practice as of how I play my clinical role on a daily basis. I keep in mind the experiences and challenges that others have gone through. However, being a Peer Support Worker and part of a great organisation, I'm aware of all of the positive movements within the services and also can see changes taking place over time. These changes are evident, which are shared within these groups, and I believe that the peer support groups illuminate hope within the members and the varying paths to recovery.

The contrast between both roles can be quite drastic. From providing one-to-one session to them working with a larger group who take the lead on fostering open discussions. This makes me sometime feel strange moving from one-to-one support to a group shared setting and helps me often find myself remembering how to switch from one role to other. This requires heightened awareness and a lot of energy at times. As a Peer Support Worker, I often examine my own stand to improve and continue to look after myself, whilst helping others on their journey. During this time, I realise that supervision is really helpful as I get to transfer my own thoughts and possibly worries to a group or during one-to-one supervision. I also attend my own counsellor regularly who has provided me with great support throughout years in my journey. At the end of a day, as both a Behavioural Therapist and a Peer Support Worker, I support myself by indulging in some self-care. After focussing whole day on others' well-being, it is important to focus on my own. Balancing both of the roles requires flexibility, compassion and a deep commitment to the well-being of clients. As I have mentioned, sometime role's confusion becomes evident, as each role has its unique challenges, different goals, approaches and professional boundaries. As a Behavioural Therapist, I uphold extra professional boundaries, whereas, in the peer support role, I'm often more open about my personal experiences and establish more informal relationships grounded on some commonality. As a Behavioural Therapist, there is a lesser level of self-disclosure as it would be deemed as less appropriate. Navigating which is appropriate in each role can be difficult at times. Learning how to balance power dynamics has also been a challenge. As a Peer Support Worker, partnerships and equality are more prevalent. Conversely, the clinician role often runs on a position of authority and expertise over the client, which can create power imbalances. The emotional burden experienced between both roles can vary also. As a Peer Support Worker, I can sometime feel more connected to client's experiences, which can often force me to reflect deeply on my personal experiences; however, in the other role, I remain more detached with a more solution-orientated mindset. In addition, balancing lived experience with professional expertise – as a Peer Support

Worker – my values stem from lived experience, but in the other role, I rely on formal education, training and clinical evidence, and balancing these two sources of knowledge can prove tricky. The balancing act can lead to internal conflict about when to share personal stories, or whether both can be merged effectively. Once the weekly peer support group is finished on the Thursday, depending upon what has been shared within the group, the next day I revisit the conversations we had and what we could pick up next week. I personally feel, I assess and analyse the peer group support more worth fully than my paid 9–5 role, with a possibility of making it more effective with passion. Working as a Peer Support Worker, I've found my role meaningful with a promise of growth and fulfilment. By sharing my experiences I've gained new meaning for past struggles and difficulties. I hope to continue to learn more about myself and others on their recovery journey and to share and understand more about myself and others in course of time.

5.3.3 Challenges from the Service/Organisation

The Peer Support Worker role also has a number of challenges to its implementation from a systemic/organisational perspective. The most prominent challenge discussed in the available literature is the ongoing biomedical culture that is still evident in services today (Ministry of Health, 1995; Smedberg, 2015; Byrne et al., 2016). The biomedical model suggests that mental health challenges are brain disorders and/or abnormalities that require pharmacological intervention to successfully treat and restore the organ back to '*normal*' functioning (Deacon, 2013). This model is in direct contradiction with the recovery model which emphasises personal responsibility, autonomy and a life worth living. This recovery model is the backbone in which peers practise within (Breslin, n.d.). In conjunction with the presence of the biomedical model comes a ripple effect which creates a risk-averse culture within the organisation (Bee et al., 2015). A risk-averse culture is one that favours coercion, restraint and containment to mitigate risk at the cost of personal autonomy and choice. Both continuous presence of the biomedical model and a culture that is risk averse demonstrate that within mental health, the service continues to lack a basic understanding of the concept of personal recovery and its related concepts, which, at times, can lead to friction (Watts et al., 2014). The friction that is present always results from the conflict observed between power and control (Byrne et al., 2015). It represents another barrier of peer support work (Blash et al., 2015). This, along with the challenges, culminates to create a toxic working environment which can often lead peers to becoming retraumatised (Migdole et al., 2011). Examples of such working environments include the unorganised setting which can retraumatise due to numerous factors, including the high acuity level, observed in service users who reside there (Smedberg, 2015). Additionally, other work environments may pose issues of stress and burnout due to poor working conditions (Moran et al., 2013; Glynn, 2023).

Stigma is another highlighted challenge from the system/organisational perspective as noted by West (2011). Blash et al. (2015) add to this, suggesting that such stigmatisation creates a rift between peer and non-peer, traditional staff. Interestingly, the source of such stigma usually stems from either the non-peer professional or the peer's practice supervisor (Smedberg, 2015). However, the peer has a duty to challenge such as stigmatising attitudes which may also cause further strife due to the '*battle*' between the peer and the traditional system. Interestingly, a lack of appropriate staff and services is also a barrier to peer support as it is impossible to implement the initiative unless the necessary physical and governance structures are in place (Byrne et al., 2017a). In addition, the friend-like relationship, introduced above and discussed in more detail in Chapter 7, is often viewed by non-peer professionals as a threat, thereby causing further friction between the peer and the various members of the MDT (Bohm et al., 2014). Another challenge identified within the available literature is the lack of recognition of the peer's source of expertise – experiential knowledge – as a viable, valuable knowledge base that can add tangibly to service provision if recognised and valued (Norton, 2024a).

In addition, a number of papers reviewed found that the peer's impact on biomedical factors and outcomes was quite poor, with some factors having no impact on the implementation of the peer into services. For instance, Boardman et al. (2014) found in their paper that the peer's impact on medication adherence was quite low. Caterlein et al. (2008) further suggest that peer interventions had little to no effect on a service user's quality of life or self-efficacy indicators. All these support a further questioning of the efficacy of peer support by traditional service providers. However, Munro et al. (2006) shed some light on this on the basis of the data presented suggesting that it is not possible to judge the implementation of peer support work into mental health service provision until the culture that currently resides within the system has changed to one resembling recovery.

5.4 Concluding Remarks

In conclusion, this chapter presented the advantages of and challenges to peer support work in mental health. From a review of the literature, it was identified that the benefits and challenges would begin at a micro (service user/Peer Support Worker) level and move gradually towards a more macro (system/organisational) level. Despite the many benefits to all stakeholders involved in the peer support initiative, there were a number of barriers – particularly towards the peer themselves and the organisation that needs addressing for peer support to survive moving forward into the future. To address these challenges, organisational and/or system level interventions are required, addressed specifically on eradicating the traditional biomedical, risk-averse culture still evident in today's services (Brown et al., 2024). In doing so, such interventions should have a mechanism of action that promotes peer values, enables role clarity and ultimately puts measures in place that makes a peer feel respected, satisfied and able to work in an effective but authentic manner (Edwards and Solomon, 2023). The following chapter starts to do this by addressing the challenges mentioned in this chapter. That is the recognition of lived experience[9] as a knowledge set that can have tremendous value to the organisation as well as to the individual service user themselves on their life-long recovery journey.

Notes

1 CHIME – Connectiveness, Hope, Identity, Meaning and purpose and Empowerment.
2 See Chapter 7 and Chapter 8.
3 See Chapter 4.
4 See Chapters 7 and Chapter 8 for more details.
5 A validated measurement used to assess a person's psychological, social and professional functioning, carried out by a physician.
6 Bed days – A term used to describe the length of stay in a hospital in treatment for a disease/injury.
7 See Chapter 6.
8 See Chapter 7 and Chapter 8 for more information on this.
9 Also known as experiential knowledge.

References

Adams, W.E. (2020) Unintended consequences of institutionalizing peer support work in mental health care. *Social Science & Medicine* 262, 113249. https://doi.org/10.1016/j.socscimed.2020.113249

Akerblom, K.B., Mohn-Haugen, T., Agdal, R. & Ness, O. (2023) Managers as peer workers' allies: A qualitative study of managers' perceptions and actions to involve peer workers in Norwegian mental health and substance use services. *International Journal of Mental Health Systems* 17, 17. https://doi.org/10.1186/s13033-023-00588-5

Austin, E., Ramakrishnan, A. & Hopper, K. (2014) Embodying recovery: A qualitative study of peer work in a consumer-run service setting. *Community Mental Health Journal* 50(8), 879–885. https://doi.org/10.1007/s10597-014-9693-z

Barlow, C.A., Schiff, J.W., Chugh, U., Rawlinson, D., Hides, E. & Leith, J. (2010) An evaluation of a suicide bereavement peer support program. *Death Studies* 34(10), 915–930. https://doi.org/10.1080/07481181003761435

Bee, P., Brooks, H., Fraser, C. & Lovell, K. (2015) Professional perspectives on service user and carer involvement in mental health care planning: A qualitative study. *International Journal of Nursing Studies* 52, 1834–1845. https://doi.org/10.1016/j.ijnurstu.2015.07.008

Beehle, M.I. & Salem, D.A. (2009) Understanding the phases of recovery from serious mental illness: The roles of referent and expert power in a mutual-help setting. *Journal of Community Psychology* 37(2), 249–267. https://doi.org/10.1002/jcop.20291

Bennetts, W., Cross, W. & Bloomer, M. (2011) Understanding consumer participation in mental health: Issues of power and change. *International Journal of Mental Health Nursing* 20(3), 155–164. https://doi.org/10.1111/j.1447-0349.2010.00719.x

Berry, C., Hayward, M.I. & Chandler, R. (2011) Another rather than other: Experiences of peer support specialist workers and their managers working in mental health services.

Journal of Public Mental Health 10(4), 238–249. https://doi.org/10.1108/1746572111 1188269

Blash, L., Chan, K. & Chapman, S. (2015) *The Peer Provider Workforce in Behavioural Health: A Landscape Analysis* (Internet). Available at: http://healthworkforce.ucsf.edu/sites/healthworkforce.ucsf.edu/files/Report-Peer_Provider_Workforce_in_Behavioral_Health-A_Landscape_Analysis.pdf (Accessed 21 December 2024).

Boardman, G., Kerr, D. & McCann, T. (2015) Peer experience of delivering a problem-solving programme to enhance antipsychotic medication adherence for individuals with schizophrenia. *Journal of Psychiatric and Mental Health Nursing* 22(6), 423–430. https://doi.org/10.1111/jpm.12195

Boardman, G., McCann, T. & Kerr, D. (2014) A peer support programme for enhancing adherence to oral antipsychotic medication in consumers with schizophrenia. *Journal of Advanced Nursing* 70(10), 2293–2302. https://doi.org/10.1111/jan.12382

Bohm, B., Glorney, E., Tapp, J., Carthy, J., Noak, J. & Moore, E. (2014) Patient focus group responses to peer mentoring in a high-security hospital. *International Journal of Forensic Mental Health* 13(3), 242–251. https://doi.org/10.1080/14999013.2014.922139

Bouchard, L., Montreuil, M. & Gros, C. (2010) Peer support among inpatients in an adult mental health setting. *Issues in Mental Health Nursing* 31, 589–598. https://doi.org/10.3109/01612841003793049

Bracke, P., Christiaens, W. & Verhaeghe, M. (2008) Self-esteem, self-efficacy and the balance of peer support among persons with chronic mental health problems. *Journal of Applied Social Psychology* 38(2), 436–459. https://doi.org/10.1111/j.1559-1816.2008.00312.x

Breslin, N. (n.d.) *Support of Peers was Key to Recovery* (Internet). Available at: www.alustforlife.com/tools/mental-health/support-of-peers-was-key-to-recovery (Accessed 23 December 2024).

Brown, L.D., Vasquez, D., Wolf, J., Robinson, J., Hartigan, L. & Hollman, R. (2024) Supporting peer support workers and their supervisors: Cluster-randomized trial evaluating a systems-level intervention. *Psychiatric Services* 75(6). https://doi.org/10.1176/appi.ps.20230112

Burke, E.M., Pyle, M., Machin, K. & Morrison, A.P. (2018) Providing mental health peer support 2: Relationships with empowerment, hope, recovery, quality of life and internal-ised stigma. *International Journal of Social Psychiatry* 64(8), 745–755. https://doi.org/10.1177/0020764018810307

Byrne, L., Happell, B. & Reid-Searl, K. (2015) Recovery as a lived experience discipline: A grounded theory study. *Issues in Mental Health Nursing* 36, 935–943. https://doi.org/10.3109/01612840.2015.1076548

Byrne, L., Happell, B. & Reid-Searl, K. (2016) Lived experience practitioners and the medical model: World's colliding? *Journal of Mental Health* 25(3), 217–223. https://doi.org/10.3109/09638237.2015.1101428

Byrne, L., Happell, B. & Reid-Searl, K. (2017a) Acknowledging rural disadvantage in mental health: Views of peer workers. *Perspectives in Psychiatric Care* 53(4), 259–265. https://doi.org/10.1111/ppc.12171

Byrne, L., Happell, B. & Reid-Searl, K. (2017b) Risky business: Lived experience mental health practice, nurses as potential allies. *International Journal of Mental Health Nursing* 26(3), 285–292. https://doi.org/10.1111/inm.12245

Cabral, L., Strother, H., Muhr, K., Sefton, L. & Savageau, J. (2014) Clarifying the role of the mental health peer specialist in Massachusetts, USA: Insights from peer specialists, supervisors and clients. *Health and Social Care in the Community* 22(1), 104–112. https://doi.org/10.1111/hsc.12072

Castelein, S., Bruggeman, R. van Busschbach, J.T., van der Gaag, M., Stant, A.D., Knegtering, H. & Wiersma, D. (2008) The effectiveness of peer support groups in psychosis: A randomized controlled trial. *Acta Psychiatrica Scandinavica* 118(1), 64–72. https://doi.org/10.1111/j.1600-0447.2008.01216.x

Chang, B-H., Mueller, L., Resnick, S.G., Osatuke, K. & Eisen, S.V. (2016) Job satisfaction of department of veteran affairs peer mental health providers. *Psychiatric Rehabilitation Journal* 39(1), 47–54. https://doi.org/10.1037/prj0000162

Cheesmond, N., Davies, K. & Inder, K.J. (2020) The role of the peer support worker in increasing rural mental health help-seeking. *Australian Journal of Rural Health* 28(2), 203–208. https://doi.org/10.1111/ajr.12603

Chinman, M., George, P., Dougherty, R.H., Daniels, A.S., Ghose, S.S., Swift, A. & Delphin-Rittmon, M.E. (2014) Peer support services for individuals with serious mental illnesses: Assessing the evidence. *Psychiatric Services* 65(4), 429–441. https://doi.org/10.1176/appi.ps.201300244

Clarke, G.N., Herinckx, H.A., Kinney, R.F., Paulson, R.I., Cutler, D.L., Lewis, K. & Oxman, E. (2000) Psychiatric Hospitalizations, arrests, emergency room visits, and homelessness of clients with serious and persistent mental illness: Findings from a randomized trial of two ACT programs vs. usual care. *Mental Health Services Research* 2(3), 155–164. https://doi.org/10.1023/A:1010141826867

Cooper, R.E., Saunders, K.R.K, Greenburgh, A., Shah, P., Appleton, R., Machin, K., Jeynes, T., Barnett, P., Allan, S.M., Griffiths, J., Stuart, R., Mitchell, L., Chipp, B., Jeffreys, S., Lloyd-Evans, B., Simpson, A. & Johnson, S. (2024) The effectiveness, implementation and experiences of peer support approaches for mental health: A systematic umbrella review. *BMC Medicine* 22, 72. https://doi.org/10.1186/s12916-024-03260-y

Davidson, L., Chinman, M., Kloos, B., Weingarten, R., Stayner, D. & Tebes, J.K. (1999) Peer support among individuals with severe mental illness: A review of the evidence. *Clinical Psychology: Science and Practice* 6, 165–187. https://doi.org/10.1093/clipsy.6.2.165

Davidson, L., Chinman, M., Sells, D. & Rowe, M. (2006) Peer support among adults with serious mental illness: A report from the field. *Schizophrenia Bulletin* 32, 443–450. https://doi.org/10.1093/schbul/sbj043

Deacon, B.J. (2013) The biomedical model of mental disorder: A critical analysis of its validity, utility, and effects on psychotherapy research. *Clinical Psychology Review* 33(7), 846–861. https://doi.org/10.1016/j.cpr.2012.09.007

Department of Health (2020) *Sharing the Vision – A Mental Health Policy for Everyone* (Internet). Available at: https://assets.gov.ie/static/documents/sharing-the-vision-a-mental-health-policy-for-everyone.pdf (Accessed 23 December 2024).

Dixon, L., Krauss, N. & Lehman, A. (1994) Consumers as service providers: The promise and challenge. *Community Mental Health Journal* 30(6), 615–625. https://doi.org/10.1007/BF02188599

Edwards, J.P. & Solomon, P.L. (2023) Explaining job satisfaction among mental health peer support workers. *Psychiatric Rehabilitation Journal* 46(3), 223–231. https://doi.org/10.1037/prj0000577

Ehrlich, C., Slattery, M., Vilic, G., Chester, P. & Crompton, D. (2020) What happens when peer support workers are introduced as members of community-based clinical mental health service delivery teams: A qualitative study. *Journal of Interprofessional Care* 34(1), 107–115. https://doi.org/10.1080/13561820.2019.1612334

Faulkner, A. & Basset, T. (2010) *A Helping Hand: Consultations with Service Users about Peer Support* (Internet). Available at: www.together- uk.org/wp-content/uploads/2023/08/A-helping-hand-consultation-with-service-users- about-peer-support.pdf (Accessed 22 December 2024).

Gillard, S., Gibson, S.L., Holley, J. & Lucock, M. (2014) Developing a change model for peer worker interventions in mental health services: A qualitative research study. *Epidemiology and Psychiatric Sciences* 24(5) 435–445. https://doi.org/10.1017/S2045796014000407

Glynn, C. (2023) *The Battle of the Peer* (Internet). Available at: https://madinireland.com/2023/05/the-battle-of-the-peer/ (Accessed 12 December 2024).

Gordon, J. & Bradstreet, S. (2015) So if we like the idea of peer workers, why aren't we seeing more? *World Journal of Psychiatry* 5(2), 160–166. https://doi.org/10.5498/wjp.v5.i2.160

Gray, B. & Sisto, M. (2024) *Peer Support in Hospital: Bridging the Gap in Mental Health* (Internet). Available at: https://pavilionhealthtoday.com/fm/peer-support-in-hospital-bridging-the-gap-in-mental-health/ (Accessed 18 December 2024).

Griffin, M. (2022) *Peer Support Working in Mental Health: A System in Need of Change* (Internet). Available at: https://madinireland.com/2022/08/peer-support-working-in-men tal-health-a-system-in-need-of-change/ (Accessed 23 December 2024).

Health Service Executive (2024) *A National Framework for Recovery in Mental Health 2024–2028* (Internet). Available at: www.hse.ie/eng/services/list/4/mental-health- ser vices/mental-health-engagement-and-recovery/resources-information-and-publications/a-national-framework-for-recovery-in-mental-health.pdf (Accessed 23 December 2024).

Hunt, E. & Byrne, M. (2019) *Peer Support Workers in Mental Health Services: A Report on the Impact of Peer Support Workers in Mental Health Services* (Internet) Available at: www.lenus.ie/bitstream/handle/10147/635104/peer-support-workers-in-mental-hea lth-services.pdf?sequence=1&isAllowed=y (Accessed 22 December 2024).

Kim, S-Y. & Kweon, Y-R. (2024) The poetry of recovery in peer support workers with mental illness: An interpretative phenomenological analysis. *Healthcare* 12(2), 123. https://doi.org/10.3390/healthcare12020123

Leamy, M., Bird, V., Le Boutillier, C., Williams, J. & Slade, M. (2011) Conceptual frame-work for personal recovery in mental health: Systematic review and narrative synthesis. *British Journal of Psychiatry* 199(6), 445–452. https://doi.org/10.1192/bjp.bp.110.083733

Meehan, T., Bergen, H., Coveney, C. & Thornton, R. (2002) Development and evaluation of a training program in peer support for former consumers. *International Journal of Mental Health Nursing* 11, 34–39. https://doi.org/10.1046/j.1440-0979.2002.00223.x

Migdole, S., Tondora, J., Silva, M.A., Barry, A.D., Milligan, J.C., Mattison, E., Rutledge, W. & Powsner, S. (2011) Exploring new frontiers: Recovery-orientated peer support pro-gramming in a psychiatric ED. *American Journal of Psychiatric Rehabilitation* 14(1), 1–12. https://doi.org/10.1080/15487768.2011.546274

Min, S-O., Whitecraft, J., Rothbard, A.B. & Salzer, M.S. (2007) Peer support for persons with co-occurring disorders and community tenure: A survival analysis. *Psychiatric Rehabilitation Journal* 30(3), 207–213. https://doi.org/10.2975/30.3.2007.207.213

Ministry of Health (1995) *A Guide to Effective Consumer Participation in Mental Health Services*. Ministry of Health, Wellington.

Miyamoto, Y. & Sono, T. (2012) Lessons from peer support among individuals with mental health difficulties: A review of the literature. *Clinical Practice and Epidemiology in Mental Health* 8, 22–29. https://doi.org/10.2174/1745017901208010022

Moll, S., Holmes, J., Geronimo, J. & Sherman, D. (2009) Work transitions for peer support providers in traditional mental health programs: Unique challenges and opportunities. *Work* 33, 449–458. https://doi.org/10.3233/WOR-2009-0893

Moran, G.S., Russinova, Z., Gidugu, V. & Gagne, C. (2013) Challenges experienced by paid peer providers in mental health recovery: A qualitative study. *Community Mental Health Journal* 49(3), 281–291. https://doi.org/10.1007/s10597-012-9541-y

Mowbray, C., Moxley, D. & Colllins, M. (1998) Consumers as mental health providers: First person accounts of benefits and limitations. *The Journal of Behavioural Health Services & Research* 25(4), 397–411. https://doi.org/10.1007/BF02287510

Mullineaux, L.M. (2017) *Service User Experiences of Peer Support in an Adult Community Mental Health Service: An Interpretative Phenomenological Analysis* (Doctor of Clinical Psychology Dissertation). University of East Anglia, United Kingdom.

Munro, K., Killoran Ross, M. & Reid, M. (2006) User involvement in mental health: Time to face up to the challenges of meaningful involvement? *International Journal of Mental Health Promotion* 8(2), 37–44. https://doi.org/10.1080/14623730.2006.9721738

Naughton, L., Collins, P. & Ryan, M. (2015) *Peer Support Workers: A Guidance Paper.* (Internet) Available at: www.hse.ie/eng/services/list/4/mental-health-services/mentalhealt hengagement/peer-support-workers-a-guidance-paper.pdf (Accessed 23 December 2024).

Norton, M.J. (2022) More than just a health care assistant: Peer support working within rehabilitation and recovery mental health services. *Irish Journal of Psychological Medicine* 23, 1–2. https://doi.org/10.1017/ipm.2022.32

Norton, M.J. (2024a) Peer work in mental health services. In *Peer Support work: Practice, Training and Implementation* (Mahon, D. ed.). Emerald Publishing Limited, Leads, pp. 9–23.

Norton, M.J. (2024b) Using learned tools for experiential gain: The application of experiential knowledge to traditional service processes. *Irish Journal of Psychological Medicine.* https://doi.org/10.1017/ipm.2024.4

Norton, M.J., Clabby, P., Coyle, B., Cruickshank, J., Davidson, G., Greer, K., Kilcommins, M., McCartan, C., McGuire, E., McGilloway, S., Mulholland, C., O'Connell-Gannon, M., Pepper, D., Shannon, C., Swords, C., Walsh, J. & Webb, P. (2023) *Peer Support Work: An International Scoping Review – Summary Report* (Internet). Available at: https://puread min.qub.ac.uk/ws/portalfiles/portal/545603311/Peer_Support_Work_Scoping_Review_ Summary_report.pdf (Accessed 22 December 2024).

O'Dwyer, O.'Brian A. (2018) *An Exploratory Study of the Peer Support Worker Role within Multi-Disciplinary Mental Health Team: Multiple Perspectives in an Irish Context* (Published Doctorate in Clinical Psychology Dissertation), University of Limerick, Limerick, Ireland.

Repper, J., Aldridge, B., Gilfoyle, S., Gillard, S., Perkins, R. & Rennison, J. (2013) *Peer Support Workers: Theory and Practice* (Internet). Available at: https://recoveryconte xtinventory.com/images/resources/ImROC_peer_support_workers_theory_practice.pdf (Accessed 22d December 2024).

Robertson, S., Leigh-Phippard, H., Roberston, D., Thomson, A., Casey, J. & Walsh, L.J. (2024) What supports the emotional well-being of peer workers in an NHS mental health service? *Mental Health and Social Inclusion.* https://doi.org/10.1108/MHSI-02-2024-0023

Roelandt, J-L., Vinet, M-A., Delissen, S., Askevis-Leherpeux, F. & Chevreul, K. (2024) Impact of follow-up by peer support workers on mental health service users' global functioning and self-stigmatisation. *L'Encephale* 50(4), 416–420. https://doi.org/10.1016/j.encep.2023.08.011

Rosenburg, D. & Argentzell, E. (2018) Service users experiences of peer support in Swedish mental health care: A "tipping point" in the care-giving culture. *Journal of Psychosocial Rehabilitation and Mental Health* 5, 53–61. https://doi.org/10.1007/s40737-018-0109-1

Saad, G., Honey, A., Schaecken, P. & Scanlan, J.N. (2024) Strategies and supports used by mental health peer workers to facilitate role performance and satisfaction. *Advances in Mental Health* 22(2), 179–195. https://doi.org/10.1080/18387357.2023.2237135

Salzer, M. & Shear, S. (2002) Identifying consumer-provider benefits in evaluations of consumer-delivered services. *Psychiatric Rehabilitation Journal* 25(3), 281–288. https://doi.org/10.1037/h0095014

Sells, D., Black, R., Davidson, L. & Rowe, M. (2008) Beyond generic support: Incidence and impact of invalidation in peer services for clients with severe mental illness. *Psychiatric Services* 59(11), 1322–1327. https://doi.org/10.1176/ps.2008.59.11.1322

Sledge, W.H., Lawless, M., Sells D., Wieland, M., O'Connell, M.J. & Davidson, L. (2011) Effectiveness of peer support in reducing readmission of persons with multiple psychiatric hospitalizations. *Psychiatric Services* 62(5), 541–544. https://doi.org/10.1176/ps.62.5.pss6205_0541

Smedberg, M.B. (2015) *The Integration of Peer Support Specialists: A Qualitative Study* (Masters of Social Work Dissertation). St Catherine University and the University of St Thomas, Minnesota, USA.

Smith, K.D. (2024) The wages of peer recovery workers: Underpaid, undervalued and unjust. *Critical Public Health* 34(1), 1–12. https://doi.org/10.1080/09581596.2024.2332796

Solomon, P. (2004) Peer support/peer guided services: Underlying processes, benefits and critical ingredients. *Psychiatric Rehabilitation Journal* 27, 392–401. https://doi.org/10.2975/27.2004.392.401

The Housing Agency (2024) *Peer Support Specialist Toolkit: Integration and Delivery of Peer Support Specialist Services* (Internet). Available at: www.housingagency.ie/sites/default/files/2024-09/The%20Housing%20Agency%20103982_Peer%20Support%20Specialist%20Toolkit_FINAL.pdf (Accessed 23 December 2024).

Trachtenberg, M., Parsonage, M., Shepherd, G. & Boardman, J. (2013) *Peer Support in Mental Health Care: Is it Good Value for Money?* (Internet). Available at: www.researchintorecovery.com/files/RRNJuly13_2013_ImROCPeersupport%20workersvalueformoney.pdf (Accessed 22 December 2024).

Tsai, A. (2002) The experiences of a "prosumer". *Psychiatric Rehabilitation Journal* 26(2), 206–207. https://doi.org/10.2975/26.2002.206.207

Walker, G. & Bryant, W. (2013) Peer support in adult mental health services: A metasynthesis of qualitative findings. *Psychiatric Rehabilitation Journal* 36(1), 28–34. https://doi.org/10.1037/h0094744

Watts, M., Downes, C. & Higgins, A. (2014) *Building Capacity in Mental Health Services to Support Recovery. An Exploration of Stakeholder Perspectives Pre and Post Intervention* (Internet). Available at: www.lenus.ie/bitstream/handle/10147/581285/ImROCIrelandReport200715.pdf?sequence=1&isAllowed=y (Accessed 22 December 2024).

West, C. (2011) Powerful choices: Peer support and individualised medication self-determination. *Schizophrenia Bulletin* 37(3), 445–450. https://doi.org/10.1093/schbul/sbp053

Part 3

Research on Peer Support Work

Chapter 6

Experiential Knowledge/Lived Experience

Case Study Contributors:

Rachael Burns and Lydia Little

6.1 Introduction

Within the last section[1] of this text, we explored the theory that is currently out there in relation to peer support work in mental health. This comprises its historical underpinnings, its definition within mental health discourse and its accompanying principles and roles along with the associated advantages and challenges. This was useful in demonstrating the current evidence base for peer support work in mental health. This present chapter marks the start of a new section within this text – one that was created to document the latest discoveries and relevant debates relating to peer support work in mental health. To do this, we start off with a chapter dedicated to the knowledge set that underpins the peer movement. It is the very thing that separates peers from non-peers. The essence can only be gathered and truly described and understood by those with lived experience of mental health challenges. This essence is known as experiential knowledge[2] – the enactment of which remains understudied at the time of writing (Kirkegaard, 2022). This is one of many such issues that this chapter aims to shed further light on.

The chapter begins in Section 6.2 where we will explore defining lived experience. This will be carried out through a critical analysis of the keywords that make up the published definitions of experiential knowledge. All of these will then be used to support the creation of a new definition for lived experience that is applicable to mental health service provision. This is followed by Section 6.3 where we will explore lived experience as a knowledge set. This involves a philosophical discussion regarding its ontological and epistemological basis in reality. After this, we will explore how lived experience as knowledge has potentially been corrupted through formalised peers being supervised by a discipline that has a different interpretation of what knowledge is and how it can be applied to that of the peer. Finally, we will explore how lived experiences are shared and the current debates around this issue. All of this leads us to Section 6.4 which offers a specific guideline regarding the authenticity of lived experience followed closely by concluding remarks in Section 6.5. Section 6.2 will now be discussed and will begin our critical analysis of this relatively new source of knowledge.

DOI: 10.4324/9781032717050-9

6.2 Defining Lived Experience

The concept of lived experience has remained ambiguous despite growing appeals to create a universal definition for the term (Parsell et al., 2024). Indeed, to this day, lived experience remains an important gap in knowledge as well as a first-hand understanding of phenomena (Carswell et al., 2022). In fact, the evidence suggests that in terms of this concept, lived experience has grown more within mental health discourse than in any other area of medicine (Davey, 2022). When we speak of lived experience, we are not describing a single, universally defined phenomenon (Hawke et al., 2022). This is because individuals who attain lived experience do so through a wide range of experiences and personal life journeys that have their own challenges, successes and personal meanings (Hawke et al., 2022). As a result, lived experience is often defined in a variety of different ways, with some lacking the precision and complexity required to move the knowledge base further along (Ajjawi et al., 2024). Additionally, there is a growing recognition of the potential value of lived experience within mental health service provision (Byrne and Wykes, 2020). As a result of this recognition, this section of the chapter aims to explore the key components of what makes a definition of lived experience to form a new definition that holds onto the desired precision and complexity required to move the knowledge base to a new level of analysis. These key components are now explored in Section 6.2.1.

6.2.1 Key Components in the Published Definitions of Lived Experience

To create a definition for lived experience, an examination of the literature occurred. What was uncovered was that, like in the process of defining peer support work,[3] although definitions varied, they all had within them several key components which proved central in the overall construction of the definition (see Table 6.1). Within this subsection of this chapter, each of these key components will be discussed in tandem below.

When I initially examined the concept of lived experience and in particular lived expertise, I knew from my own lived experiences that it was formed through the combination of the experience of the mental ill health/recovery journey and other factors arising from the social world (see Figure 6.1) (Byrne and Roennfeldt, 2024). However, through an in-depth analysis of lived experience through the available literature, I uncovered that there are far more elements at play than I originally realised (see Table 6.1). What follows is an attempt to synthesise the above key components into a comprehensive, new definition, which will inform the remainder of this text.

The first key component relevant to the concept of lived experience is that of the **experience** itself (Global Mental Health Peer Network, n.d.; Health Service Executive, 2024a, 2024b; Hyde, 2017; National Suicide Research Foundation, 2024; Office of Mental Health Engagement and Recovery, 2023; World Health

Table 6.1 Key Components in Defining Lived Experience

No.	Key Component	Explanation
1.	**Experience**	Of directly experiencing mental health difficulties/witnessing a loved one as they experience mental health difficulties.
		Of utilising mental health services.
		Of the impact of the above two factors on a person's life.
		Of managing one's mental health either periodically or on an ongoing basis.
2.	**A Journey**	Encompasses the entire person's journey from the beginning of a person's recovery journey[4] till the end of life.
3.	**Expertise**	The insight and knowledge that can only be attained from living through a mental health challenge.
4.	**Value**	Lived experience has both a therapeutic and service improvement value.
5.	**Subjective, Unique and Personal**	Lived experience is a subjective, unique and personalised experience for everyone regardless of role[5]
6.	**Recollection**	Requires the individual to recall events, traumas, emotional and cognitive processes and other circumstances relevant to the experience of mental ill health.
7.	**Epistemological Significance and Phenomenological Richness of Personal Narratives**	Recognising the underlying importance of the personal narrative in shaping one's perception of reality.
		The experience, although different for everyone, is full of knowledge about the person's inner and social worlds.
8.	**Interplay**	Between one's subjective interpretations, their emotions and contextual factors that all make up a person's mental health journey.
9.	**Knowledge**	Recognising these experiences as a valid form of knowledge.
10.	**Catalyst**	For change and transformation for all societal systems.
11.	**Deep Listening**	So that the support offered responds to both the causes and consequences of social and structural determinants.

Individual Experiences	➕	Collective Impacts and Identification	🟰	Lived Expertise
Describes: impacts of life-changing individual experiences, including: types of service use or inability to access services, and impacts of intersectionality		Describes: common impacts of adversity as a result of lived experience, and identification within the peer community		Describes: learnt mastery - individual experiences and collective impacts being understood, and that understanding utilised to assist others
Knowledge/abilities gained Deep, personal understanding of particular types of individual experience. The ability to connect over 'like' or similar experiences, including more marginalised experiences and identities		**Knowledge/abilities gained** Challenging stigma by publicly identifying as having a lived experience. Ability to connect over and represent common impacts of adversity, trauma, marginalisation, stigma etc. Connection to the wider peer community and/or alignment with collective thinking		**Demonstrated knowledge/abilities** Articulate the impacts of adverse experiences and how life/concept of self has changed. Highly developed relational skills, including advanced use of empathy and effective sharing of personal recovery story. Understanding how essential hope is, strategies to build hope, and holding hope for others. Redefining experiences in a way that is empowering and helpful – transforming adversity to expertise. Understanding and articulating how peer work is distinct and unique, including peer values, principles and practice

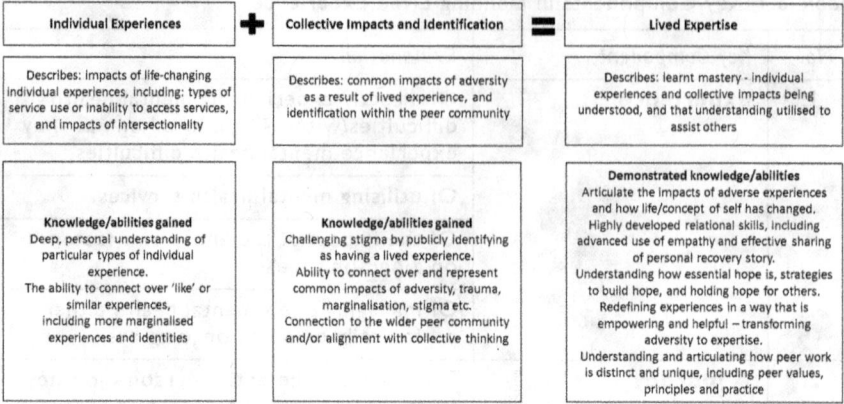

Figure 6.1 Factors Required for the Creation of Lived Expertise.

Organisation, 2019). However, the experience itself is multifaceted and is not just about directly experiencing or witnessing a loved one as they experience a mental health difficulty (Health Service Executive, 2024a, 2024b; Hyde, 2017; National Suicide Research Foundation, 2024; Office of Mental Health Engagement and Recovery 2023). Indeed, it also involves the specific use of mental health services to restore mental well-being (Global Mental Health Peer Network, n.d.; Health Service Executive, 2024a, 2024b), as well as the impact of both factors on a person's life (Global Mental Health Peer Network, n.d.; Health Service Executive, 2024a; Hyde, 2017; World Health Organisation, 2019). When we discuss impacts, we mean more than a direct impact from the use of services and the illness itself. Impacts are also noted as being related to concepts that are social and human-rights-based – for example discrimination, epistemic injustice, stigmatisation, coercion and ostracisation. Finally, experiences also refer to the management of one's mental health challenges either periodically or on an ongoing basis (Health Service Executive, 2024b).

These experiences noted above suggest that the actor travels through each of these sets of experiences over the course of **a journey** that has been noted as life-long (Health Service Executive, 2024b) Such experiences are said to have both a therapeutic and service improvement **value** (Health Service Executive, 2023). Valuing these perspectives allows them to become a knowledge set with particular **expertise** that can only derive from living through mental health challenges (Goulding et al., 2024). Such expertise also allows for the traditional system to be challenged to foster a more profound understanding of mental health (Goulding et al., 2024). The experience is also **unique** (Goulding et al., 2024; Health Service Executive, 2023; Global Mental Health Peer Network, n.d.; Office of Mental Health Engagement and Recovery 2023), **subjective** (Goulding et al., 2024) and **personalised** (Office of Mental Health Engagement and Recovery 2023) to each individual regardless of role within the system.

Lived experience goes beyond the generation of knowledge and skills (Global Mental Health Peer Network, n.d.). Instead, it's a **recollected** approach that is influenced by traumas, emotive and cognitive processes and other circumstances relevant to the experience of mental ill health (Office of Mental Health Engagement and Recovery 2023). Indeed, it requires an acknowledgement of the **epistemological significance and phenomenological richness of the personal narrative** in shaping one's reality and indeed one's social world (Goulding et al., 2024; Ridley et al., 2024). In this way, lived experience allows one to focus attention on the realities and pains that are created by our own social realities – for instance poverty to war, famine, racism and colonial histories (Montague-Cardoso et al., 2024). In this way lived experience has multiple dilemmas which require an individual to **interplay** between subjective interpretations and emotional as well as contextual factors that shape one's narrative and subsequent journey (Goulding et al., 2024). Through this interplay, the **knowledge** that is subsequently created acts as a **catalyst** for transformation and change that impacts all societal systems (Global Mental Health Peer Network, n.d.; Owen et al., n.d.). Finally, this resulting knowledge supports the Peer Support Worker to engage in active, critical and **deep listening** during their time with service users so that the support offered by the peer can respond to both the causes and consequences of issues within the service user's social world (Montague-Cardoso et al., 2024).

6.2.2 A Definition of Lived Experience to Be Used in This Text

As identified above, the concept of lived experience has been observed to have several components that are key to defining it. Now that this has been explored, these components have been placed together to construct a new, novel definition for the term. From which the following definition was constructed suggesting that, lived experience in mental health is:

> *A knowledge set that involves the recollection of subjective, unique and personal experiences that are epistemologically significant and phenomenologically rich with that of other experiences and expertise that are gathered and that interplay with one another throughout the life journey which provide both a therapeutic and service improvement value by acting as a catalyst for deep, critical listening and reflection so that peers can respond to issues that arise within one's social world.*

However, the above is a technical, somewhat jargon-filled definition for something that is simple but transformative. In the following case study, Rachael explores what lived experience is for her – identifying from her experience as a peer a number of important elements central to the creation of lived experience, to that knowledge set that is truly transformative.

Case Study 5   The Most Valuable Asset

Rachael Burns

Anyone (given adequate intellect, enough money, hard work, and other aligning circumstances) can attain a degree. That is not to say that it is an easy feat – it certainly is not! However, it has become quite a common possession across many fields and serves as a foundation for many professionals. Whilst jumping through the hoops of courses and certifications is still often a necessity in the peer space, it is not the primary qualification. Rather, it is **lived experience** – a personal level of understanding far beyond what can be laid out by a set curriculum. Textbooks and articles and academic titles only account for so much. Reality cannot be summarised into chapters and organised into units that neatly span the course of a semester. It cannot be captured in words and preserved in its integrity, nor can it be understood and comprehended in its entirety. Knowledge that is manufactured holds value, for sure, but it is only one piece of a much more expansive puzzle.

I have Lived Experience with many mental illnesses. I have lost years to Anorexia Nervosa, comorbid with Obsessive Compulsive Disorder, Major Depressive Disorder, Generalised Anxiety Disorder, Complex Post-Traumatic Stress Disorder and more. These diagnoses are not my identity, but they contribute largely to the person that I am today. However, at many points in my treatment, clinicians have treated me as though they were. To me it was always glaringly obvious what was intellectualised. What was boiled down to a two-dimensional description of a disorder. I have always been able to discern what lines are memorised as opposed to spoken from the heart. Whilst delivered with all the greatest intention, they feel patronising and infantilising. Contrastingly, there is something so dignifying about someone carrying their own personal experience, heart, and vulnerabilities from a place of non-judgement and mutuality. Which in itself strips away the clinical jargon and steps outside of psychoanalysis, instead drawing from the commonality that unites us all, basic humanity.

Perhaps the only times I've truly been seen, validated, accepted, and TRULY accommodated have been in this space. Certainly, in my own recovery, the value of lived experience cannot be understated. Admittedly still in the process of finding who I am and healing my wounds into scars, peer work has been and is still a North Star. Lived experience practice adds another layer to healing – one that many don't get to encounter – to use pain for something positive. That is not to justify or accept the things that should never have been true, but to use them as tools that can be shared with those still fighting. Navigating this as a career is another challenge entirely. It comprises numerous skills coming together in unison, some of the most valuable of these being as follows:

Acknowledgement to Country and of Lived Experience

I am an Australian of European ancestry, who sits writing on and in Boorloo, Whadjuk Noongar Boodja. I pay my respects to elders past, present, and emerging. I hold deep regard for the cultural practices and Dreamtime legends that made this country the breathtaking and sacred place I am fortunate enough to call home. Australia was, is, and always will be stolen land. Built on years of genocide and dehumanising apartheid. Of disregard for culture and violation of human rights, of stigma and hostility and hardship. It is essential that upon every instance, this is acknowledged and attributed.

Similarly, it is essential to acknowledge the value and weight of lived experience that sits within a room. The endless unique and diverse perspectives that come together in a peer environment, in which each person brings value simply by being present. It is equally as important to acknowledge the strength shown by those who fight mental illness every day, those who have pathed the way in the revolution that is the consumer movement, those lost along the way, and those who walk alongside.

Safe Sharing

As people with lived experience, our words and stories are powerful. They are our truth. One that cannot be denied and should not have to be diluted for others' comfort. However, when working with people that themselves are vulnerable, boundaries are an essential safeguard. What we say can have beneficial power, without argument, but there is also a potential for detriment. Intimate details, numbers, measurements, and imagery can not only be distressing to hear, but it can also provide a bar for unhelpful comparison. We – as peers – have a responsibility to share meaningfully and safely. This in itself is ill-defined. What is regarded as '*safe*' cannot be determined by a blanket rule, and will vary in different situations.

In my case, there are boundaries that I will not cross. Eating disorders – anorexia especially – are very competitive, and going into the intimate details will **never** be helpful – ESPECIALLY not for those actively struggling or in recovery. I will never share numbers – weight, calories, admission number, Body Mass Index (BMI) … you name it. I will also never share graphic depictions such as photos or explicit stories. I will never delve into the details of my most distressing traumas nor will I share '*before and after*' comparisons. Not only is this out of good conscience to protect others and myself, it is also my *duty* as a person sharing my story publicly. Narratives of this type reinforce harmful stereotypes which prevent many from seeking help. This primarily pertains to Eating Disorders and the idea that people who experience them (anorexia in particular) are underweight and that the degree of suffering correlates to their physicality. This is simply not true – a person can be struggling immensely at any weight/shape. In fact only 6% of people with eating disorders are medically underweight (ANAD, 2023[4]). Anyone sharing their story has the responsibility to do so safely and – by extension – in a manner that does not reinforce stereotypes.

Multiple Truths and Individuality

As humans, it is natural to hold strong convictions. To believe that *our* way of seeing things is *the* way of seeing things, and that any other perspective is inherently incorrect. *Our* truth is indeed *the* truth viewed through the lens of all of our own past experiences and thought processes. It's important to recognise that each individual has their own life experiences, vexes, and (sometimes distortive) lenses, thus knowing a different ultimate truth. This may not necessarily align with our own, and that's okay. The goal in working with peers is to make it safe to hold differing opinions and to acknowledge these without judgement, and to best accommodate the unique preferences of individuals.

Caveats

Using and sharing lived experience should also be met with relevant caveats at each separate instance. Some of the caveats that I find myself frequenting thinking about are as follows:

- Although my story includes periods of hospitalisation, this is not a requirement and does not make my experience any more or less than another person's.
- Although my eating disorder very much played into the stereotypical image of anorexia, this is a small minority. The severity of someone's suffering does not correlate to a physicality.
- Although something may be merely uncomfortable for one person, the same experience may be perceived as traumatic for another person. This is not a reflection of '*weakness*' rather it is a testament to individuality.

Accepting that We Can Never FULLY Understand

Whilst two people may have *similar* experiences, no two people will ever have *the same* experience. Something I've noticed is that people have a tendency to comfort others by claiming they fully relate, but this in itself can be deeply invalidating – even when done so amongst peers. Certainly, peers often have an ability to relate at a level deeper than every-day folk, they still will never comprehend one's experiences in their entirety. This is okay. It is expected. It is human. It is also something that we should not attempt to do, as it reduces the complex experiences of another that are shaped by various different lenses, genetics, upbringings, and lives to something trivial. It compresses the three-dimensionality of the human experience into something plain.

Social Awareness

Working in and existing in the peer space is something that not everyone is suited for. It requires an ability to read the room and tune into silent signals. To pick up on subtleties and know how to address them. To understand the difference between listening to speak and listening to hear, and knowing the value of silence. Of course, a degree of this can be learned, but I believe it is more so an inherent skill held by only a small margin of the population. Peers need a high degree of social awareness accompanied by compassion, wisdom and skill.

Keeping the 'greater good' in Mind

I don't believe that people who experience mental illness 'owe' anything to the world, however I do believe that there is a debt to be repaid to the past versions of ourselves, to those no longer with us, and to those still unable to find a voice. In times where peer work becomes heavy and disempowering, this is something that is valuable to keep in mind and to use as a driver.

Power of Choice

Mental illness is not a choice, and for many of us treatment pillages a lot of our autonomy and ability to make decisions pertaining to our own health. Many people who have been treated as a psychiatric patient know what it is like to be devoid of choice, especially those who have been treated involuntarily. As such, it is infinitely reassuring and empowering to ensure that at every opportunity possible they are provided with choice.

Reclaiming Terminology

Given the traumatic nature of psychiatric treatment, many of the terms and jargon that comes alongside it carries very negative and frightening connotations for those who have experienced it. Not only this, a lot of the terminology that is used is either outdated, devalued after being thrown around, simplistic, or demeaning to certain people. To me, the term *'recovery'* is a prime example of this. It is something that has been thrown around and devalued. That has been used as a threat and that many have tried to force upon me, this the word in itself has negative associations. For me, it also doesn't align at a deeper level. To me, *'recovery'* denotes an endpoint. It feels so final, a reversion to one's past self in a sense. Ignorance towards the life-changing experiences of illness and denial at a core level. Having said this, recovery is a term that is widely used and understood. For many, it does hold hope. Even though it isn't my preference, it may be for others and thus I must put aside my own personal beliefs. Peer work – fundamentally – is not about catering to my preferences, it is about those of the people I work with. It is ***their*** time and ***their*** space.

Comfort

I've definitely noticed the importance of comfort, and the barrier constructed when this is denied. It makes a world of difference to take into account a person's small preferences. Things like where a conversation takes place, who is in the room, what supports are available, lighting, noise levels, and smells that may be present. What seems like such a small detail to many medically trained practitioners is something so major to individuals and something that peers have the ability to accommodate.

Owning Mistakes

Being human is facing the reality that we often get things wrong. No matter how much restraint, how much skill and how much care we take, it is bound to happen. The key to good practice is not the absence of mistakes, rather the ability to accept, make amends, and move forward.

The field of Lived Experience as a whole is beautiful when navigated with due care. The way in which the learned knowledge of fellow human beings bridges gaps that the medical and psychiatric fields both cannot is nothing short of incredible. It now brings me great pride to share that I am a person with lived experience of mental illness. Something that I once buried underneath piles of lies and deceit that now stands tall. I truly believe that lived experience is the key to meaningful, lasting change, and I am honoured to be a part of this movement.

As Rachael so eloquently presents, lived experience is unique and different for everyone. In this text alone, Rachael, I and the many sources referenced in this book all present lived experiences in a different way based on our own experiences.

We are all right from our own perspective. However, with the creation of this new definition for lived experience, brought about through the synthesis of several key texts, we can now begin to observe the simplicity and complexity of lived experience as a knowledge set within mental health discourse.

6.3 Lived Experience as a Knowledge Set

Now that we have a new understanding of what is termed '*lived experience*', it is now time to examine several areas that are of current interest in both its application and practice. We begin this journey in Section 6.3.1 where experiential knowledge as a knowledge set in its own right will be philosophically examined so that its ontological and epistemological positioning can be determined. This is followed by Section 6.3.2 which will look at the attempts of non-peers to corrupt the essence of lived experience in peer support practice. Of particular interest here are the current governance and supervisory relationships of the peer – with examples from an Irish context given to support the explanation. Finally, Section 6.3.3 will end our exploration into current interest issues by examining the current debates regarding the sharing of lived experiences within peer support work. Given the transformative power lived experience – particularly its workforce – has for mental health service provision, the issues that will be discussed here are of significance if we are to progress this source of knowledge and transformation further (Australian Government National Mental Health Commission, 2023).

6.3.1 Ontological and Epistemological Positioning of Lived Experience

Ontology as a philosophical concept is used and defined differently depending on what context one is situated within (Guarino et al., 2009). In this text, we will refer to Stichbury's conceptualisation of the term which states simply that ontology is a mechanism of describing the world based on several factors including relationships. (Stichbury, 2017). In this way, it refers to an understanding of what reality is (Ylonen and Aven, 2023). Epistemology on the other hand is intrinsically linked to that of ontology but differs as it explores how we come to know something is in truth or reality (Kivunja and Kuyini, 2017). Simply put, epistemology centres on the creation and observation of knowledge within the realms of multiple realities. Some work has already been carried out on exploring the philosophical basis of experiential knowledge, mainly centred around the social sciences. Within healthcare, Dumez and L'Esperance (2024) have explored theoretically experiential knowledge where they suggest that experiential knowledge can be divided into six types of patient knowledge which can work together to create the knowledge set that we know as experiential (see Figure 6.2).

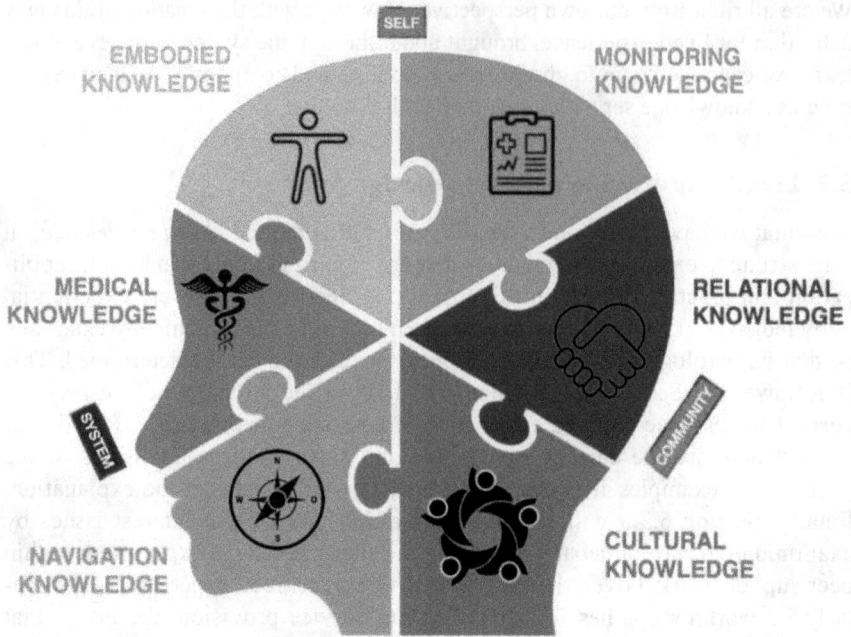

Figure 6.2 Six Types of Patient Knowledge.

These six types of patient knowledge are used to broaden the understanding of experiential knowledge in health care and are based on the experiences acquired through the self, the system and the community (Dumez and L'Esperance, 2024). They are further examined in Table 6.2.

Taking these six types of patient knowledge under consideration, it is clear that experiential knowledge does not sit within the realm of positivism. Indeed, a recently commissioned report by Goulding et al. (2024) suggests that experiential knowledge is an intricate and multi-layered concept which shifts away from a positivist notion towards valuing subjective understanding. As such, experiential knowledge is interpretive in nature as this ontological stance allows for multiple subjective understandings of reality. An important distinction to make to that of biomedical knowledge which suggests there is only one observable and measurable truth or reality. Identifying an epistemological stance for experiential knowledge is not an easy feat. As noted in Dumez and L'Esperance (2024)'s empirical paper, the knowledge that makes up lived experience does not come from just one source – as is often debated within other disciplines. Instead, experiential knowledge involves the interplay of all six aspects of patient knowledge which work together to help the peer identify their social world, what is in it and how they can use their experiences in this world to support themselves and others in their respective recovery journeys. As such, given the above, it is fair to assume that lived experience is

Table 6.2 Explained – Six Types of Patient Knowledge

No.	Type of Patient Knowledge	Explanation
1.	**Embodied Knowledge**	Sensory, grounded on physical bodily experience like pain as well as psychologically orientated perceptions. Vulnerabilities and bodily strengths become signs that individuals listen to and use to make decisions
2.	**Monitoring Knowledge**	Describes the capacity of individuals to identify signs and symptoms of acuity in one's physical, mental and/or emotional health. Through a recognition of signs and symptoms of deteriorating health, individuals are able to make decisions based on bodily, sensory, physical and psychological manifestations.
3.	**Navigation Knowledge**	Acquired from the repeated use of health services and repeated institutional access and subsequent barriers to healthcare. Here, the individual utilises these repeated experiences to ensure they have the most efficient access to necessities and benefits.
4.	**Medical Knowledge**	Have an understanding of medical language and can initiate conversations about their illness, their care and treatment. Used by peers to bargain a position of credibility to make sense of their illness.
5.	**Relational Knowledge**	A form of situated knowledge that allows individuals to know who to contact within their community to access a particular service. It is about knowing the role each actor of the MDT plays within one's care.
6.	**Cultural Knowledge**	Inclusive of cultural norms, values symbols and constructs that make up a social world that subsequently influences the experience of life and illness. Here, this type of patient knowledge not only refers to the cultural codes in the social world but also how they influence how one conceptualises and makes preferences surrounding health, treatment and care relationships.

Source: Extracted from Dumez and L'Esperance (2024).

constructed rather than observably evident in the social world. Equally, it is not a theoretical concept – but an actual fusion of multiple sources of knowledge within the social world. Each actor within this world must build their own understanding of the world in different ways and no two are ever the same. Hence leading to the suggestion that no experience is truly observed in the same way. Additionally, reality is not already present upon entry into a social world – as is believed in positivist ontological stances. Rather the actor within the social world must build or construct their reality based on the tools and techniques they manifest through the application of Dumez and L'Esperance's six types of patient knowledge in the social world. As such, in conclusion, experiential knowledge has an **interpretive ontology** with an associated **social constructionist epistome**.

6.3.2 Corruption of Lived Experience by the Non-Peer Professional

Globally, an emphasis has developed placing importance on the inclusion of lived experience within all aspects of mental health service provision (Sunkel and Sartor, 2022). However, the meaningful integration of lived experience within such settings has faced several challenges (Speyer et al., 2024; Sunkel and Sartor, 2022). One such area in which this has arisen is that of supervision and more broadly the governance structures related to the role (Norton et al., 2023).

Firstly, we will examine the idea of the corruption of lived experience through supervision. Supervision in peer support is defined as a collaborative relationship between the Peer Support Worker and their supervisor (Watson et al., 2024). Given that operating as a Peer Support Worker brings with it its own unique challenges,[6] it is essential that peers receive regular and ongoing supervision whilst actively engaging in the role (Health Service Executive, n.d.). Within Irish mental health services, the supervision of peers centres around the Morrison's (2005) 4×4×4 model – a model commonly used in social work and now adapted to aid in the supervision of peers (Mahon and Norton, 2024). In other jurisdictions, specific frameworks have been developed to support the activity of peer supervision. For example, the Australia-based Lived Experience Workforce Program (2019) has developed a framework to aid peer supervision. This framework is not in isolation from the United States Bureau of Justice Assistance (2022), also developing a toolkit of its own to support the same.

Within an Irish context, supervision and line management duties – at the time of writing –currently are undertaken by the profession of social work (Mahon and Norton, 2024). The supervision of peers by non-peers is not only noted in an Irish context, with many peer supervisors in the United States being from the non-peer mental health service provider cohort (Forbes and Pratt, 2019). According to Norton and colleagues, there are two main ways in which non-peer staff can corrupt or negatively impact the integrity of the Peer Support Worker role. These include the lack of role clarity and the imposition of non-peers onto the peer's knowledge set and subsequent epistemological position (Norton et al., 2023). As already discussed, a lack of role clarity is an extreme challenge to peer support work in mental health on a number of different levels (Hunt and Byrne, 2019). This is despite the expansive amount of literature exploring peer support work that is currently available. This as alluded to by Norton and colleagues, threatens the unique insider position held by these workers. In terms of imposing an epistemological position, according to Norton et al. (2023), this occurs when due to power imbalances between the supervisor and the peer, as well as a lack of clarity on behalf of the supervisor as to the peer role, peers may be conformed to a way of working that is not conducive of or authentic to that of lived experience.

Peer support work is not just being corrupted at a micro, individualised level. It also is corrupted at a mesosystem and organisational level. Taking Irish mental health services as an example, there has not, until recently, been a confirmed governance structure in place for Peer Support Workers (see Figure 6.3).

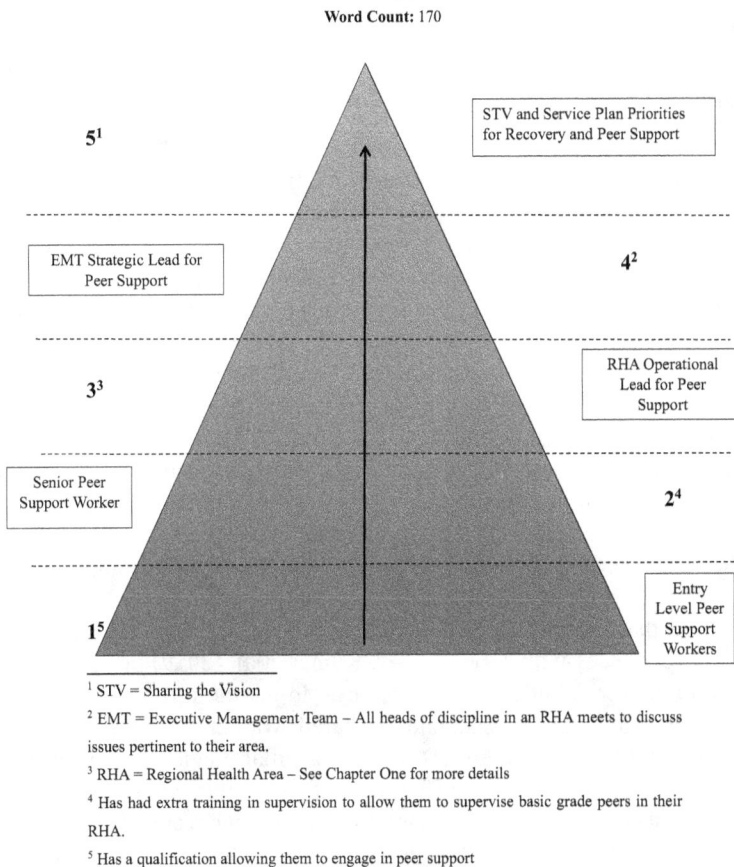

Word Count: 170

5[1] — STV and Service Plan Priorities for Recovery and Peer Support

EMT Strategic Lead for Peer Support — **4[2]**

3[3] — RHA Operational Lead for Peer Support

Senior Peer Support Worker — **2[4]**

1[5] — Entry Level Peer Support Workers

[1] STV = Sharing the Vision

[2] EMT = Executive Management Team – All heads of discipline in an RHA meets to discuss issues pertinent to their area.

[3] RHA = Regional Health Area – See Chapter One for more details

[4] Has had extra training in supervision to allow them to supervise basic grade peers in their RHA.

[5] Has a qualification allowing them to engage in peer support

Figure 6.3 Peer Support Worker Governance Structure.

As noted in Figure 6.3, in terms of governance, the Peer Support Worker follows a chain of command that stretches from the micro (individualised level) to the meso (organisational level) and finally to that of the macro (governmental/national level). In terms of Irish services, the corruption comes from both service readiness as well as career progression issues. At the time of writing, Senior Peer Support Workers are yet to be recruited, causing much frustration within the peer community. In addition, the specialised training in supervision that is required for senior peers has yet to be commissioned. Finally, and most challenging of all is that this governance structure – at the time of writing – has only been agreed upon in certain Regional Health Areas, with a number yet to confirm commitment to the structure. None of this is helped by the structural reform that is taking place as a direct result of Slaintecare[7] (2017), which indeed also threatens the future development of this new resource within health services. Given this multi-level corruption of lived experience, addressing the same will require the use of an organisational/system-wide approach (Brown et al, 2024). Such strategies will be discussed later in Section 6.4.

6.3.3 Sharing Lived Experience – Current Debates

Within peer support work, the appropriate application of lived experience is observed as an essential element in the recovery of those with mental health problems (Parr, 2023; Simmons et al., 2023). Through the sharing of lived experience, an in-depth understanding of life from the perspective of those who have experienced mental distress themselves is uncovered which has been shown to have therapeutic properties (Colori, 2021; Uren and Inder, 2021). Within peer support work, lived experience is shared for three central reasons: (1) to normalise an individual's experiences, (2) to develop a mutual, non-hierarchical space we call informality[8] and (3) to identify the Peer Support Worker as a role model for the recipient of such experiences to follow (Norton, 2022, 2023). Additionally, sharing lived experiences is an important practice because it is through this process that learning regarding one's own mental health can begin to occur (Eronen, 2019).

Despite the benefits of sharing lived experiences, as suggested by Norton (2022, 2023), there have been challenges and barriers that have limited its appropriate use within services (Reeves et al., 2024). Indeed, a recent chapter by Norton (2024) has suggested that there remains much debate regarding how one should share their lived experiences with service users. Kumar et al. (2019) begin this debate by suggesting that in order for the service user to get the full benefit from lived experience, the whole narrative should be shared. Wall et al. (2022) highlight an issue in sharing the entire narrative – that of a similar diagnosis. However, Wall and colleagues do suggest that the sharing of the narrative can still be effective, despite differences in diagnosis. Similar findings were uncovered by Lessard et al. (2024) who noted that it is not the similarity in diagnosis that is of therapeutic value, rather it is the sharing of hardships that can only be adequately demonstrated through the sharing of the entire narrative that is of value as it is through these shared hardships that true connections that are therapeutic can occur. Thomson and Balaam (2020) add to this conversation by suggesting that when a peer goes about sharing their personal narrative, they need to remember that the service user needs are of primary concern and as such the narrative may need to be modified to ensure that what is shared is of therapeutic value to the service user and less so the peer.

This idea of sharing the entire narrative within peer support work is not shared by all who write about this particular act in peer support work. According to Bailie (2015) and Mullineaux (2017), the sharing of lived experiences should be limited to what is similar between the peer and the recipient service user. Truong et al. (2019) add to this debate by suggesting that the sharing of lived experiences should not focus on the peer's experiences, but instead what is shared should be somewhat relevant to the recipient service user's own situational context. Similar findings are identified by Change Mental Health (n.d.) that suggests that the crux of sharing lived experiences is to identify similarities in terms of the person's struggles and use that to provide comfort. Within a blog post, Glynn (2023) describes how she shared similarities when utilising lived experience in her role. Such sharing creates meaningful connections that ultimately allow for emotional healing to occur (Glynn, 2023). As will be discussed in the forthcoming chapter,[9] the purpose of sharing lived experience is to create a mutual and equal relationship. However, to do this, there needs to be similarities in what is being shared, specifically relating to one's demographics and/or social standing (Penny, 2018). Thoits (2021) adds to this suggesting that the similarities that should be shared between the peer and the recipient service user should centre around one or more social statuses along with the experience of distress.

Interestingly, according to Archard et al. (2023), the disclosure of lived experience within peer support roles is not as prominent as what management and policy makers originally anticipated. However, in the absence of a clear consensus as to what should be shared and when, it is essentially up to the Peer Support Worker to decide what they wish to share and when, based on what they are comfortable with sharing and what is of therapeutic value to the service user they are working with (Kennedy and Mead, 2019).

6.4 Guideline – Protecting the Authenticity of Lived Experience

Authentic peer support work is extremely important for the personal recovery of service users (Gruhl et al., 2015). Within mental health discourse, peer support work is said to be authentic if it meets three conditions: (1) if the peer can draw on their lived experience as a source of knowledge, (2) if the peer can engage in meaningful discussions with the recipient service user regarding personal recovery and (3) if the peer can be identified and act as a role model for the service users they work with (Gruhl et al., 2015). However, to meet these conditions of authenticity, adequate supervision of the peer is vital (Repper et al., 2013). However, it has been reported that in recent years, organisations that have implemented peers have raised concerns over contradictory supervision practices that conflict with the core values of peer support work[10] (Foglesong et al., 2021). Such practices pose a significant challenge in implementing and sustaining such roles within mental health settings (Cooeyate et al., 2024).

Additionally, the lack of career progression for peers is a noted barrier to the authenticity of peer support work as there are no structures in place to support peer supervision. This is an important remark as supervision of the peer with non-peer professionals presents a hierarchy that is not conducive to the core principles and values of peer support work (Norton, 2023). Within an Irish setting, the best approach to counteracting this issue is to create a new grade of peer support work that has responsibility for the supervision of basic grade peers. These Senior Peer Support Workers would ensure that supervision remains mutual but is also representative of peer values (see Appendix for a copy of the job specification for the role of Senior Peer Support Worker). However, in their absence, guidelines should be developed to support either external peer supervisors or non-peer supervisors in the supervision of Peer Support Workers (Castles et al., 2023). Such guidelines (see Table 6.3) should be included in training given to non-peer supervisors to support them in becoming peer allies and champions within mental health discourse until such time as the Senior Peer Support Worker role is rolled out in mental health service provision (Plante, 2024).

In our next case study, Lydia highlights the unique challenges and rewards of supervising peers in a peer-led service within the NHS, whilst also highlighting areas for consideration in the supervision of such employees.

6.5 Concluding Remarks

There is now a global consensus that those with lived experience hold a certain type of knowledge that plays a particularly important role in influencing policy and practices at a global scale (Sartor, 2023). Within mental health services, Peer Support Workers – no matter where they are based – require lived experience of mental health challenges and service use (either their own or as a carer) to function correctly and connect with others in the community they serve (Roberson et al., 2024). This chapter focussed on the knowledge set created by lived experience: experiential knowledge – to explore the same in depth ranging from a philosophical level all the way through to its practical application by Peer Support Workers within mental health service provision. As we move forward, continued recognition of the power of lived experience in shaping both policy and practice is needed in order for peer roles to flourish within such environments (Marshall et al., 2024).

Table 6.3 Guidelines for Non-Peer Supervisors in the Supervision of Peer Support Workers

	Model A	*Model B*
Supervision Arrangement	Peer Support Workers are supervised (administrative and supportive) by a supervisor on the MDT[11]	Peer Support Workers are supervised (administrative and supportive) by a supervisor on the MDT. The Area Engagement Lead[12] or someone within the HSE[13] with lived experience in mental health provides coaching/ mentoring and training to peers in their area.
Frequency and Structure of 1:1 Peer Support Specific Supervision	Monthly (minimum), flexible to accommodate needs. Is combined with administrative supervision (discussing performance and work plan)	Monthly supervision from MDT. Supervisory and ongoing mentoring ranges from twice monthly to once every two months. This may be individual or in groups depending on capacity.
	Additional supervision needs to be provided by all supervisors if Peer Support Workers are struggling, returning from leave or facing changes in their work.	
	Discussions of • Relationships with colleagues • Workplace culture • Using lived experience • Core peer support practices • Reflective practice • Self-care and workplace wellness strategies • Boundaries • Navigating conflict • Opportunities to strengthen lived experience voices	
New Peer Support Workers to the HSE	Includes shadowing in a peer support service for several days Includes training the interdisciplinary team on peer support philosophy, history, and practices related to supervising Peer Support Workers Includes in-depth training for Peer Support Workers on core practices of peer support working.	

(Continued)

Table 6.3 (Continued)

	Model A	Model B
Benefits and Risks	All supervisors need defined role/strong role clarity and good communication between supervisors and mentors. Model B can lead to over-supervision and a risk of triangulation between Peer Support Workers and their supervisors. When implemented well both models help Peer Support Workers feel supported and confident in their roles. Model B allows for the Peer Support Worker to align themselves to others with lived experience and keep true to the role.	

Source: Adapted from Health Service Executive (n.d.).

Note: There are two proposed models of supervision recommended for Peer Support Workers, depending on service preference and/or need.

Case Study 6   Managing a Peer Team in Traditional Services

Lydia Little

Managing a team of lived experience and peer staff brings unique challenges and rewards, requiring a different approach than traditional management structures. Here, I will discuss how peer management holds at its core a type of leadership which focuses on creating an environment of ontological security – a state of mental well-being where team members feel a deep sense of stability, trust, and psychological safety. As a manager, fostering this environment is not just about supporting employees professionally; it is about respecting and validating their personal experiences, emotional responses, and the insights they bring to the table.

The guiding ethos I use was originally co-created by my staff team in a peer crisis house situated in the third sector, the first known team of its kind in England. This ethos ensured that everyone contributed their voice in how we worked together, and which values guide our day-to-day interactions. This ethos is built on five central tenets that were collaboratively agreed upon, creating a foundation of mutual respect, and understanding and I hope that you find this useful when considering future projects – regardless of your level of seniority or input.

Relationships Are Everyone's Responsibility

One of the first principles we established as a team was the shared responsibility for maintaining relationships. In a typical workplace, relationship management is often assumed to be the responsibility of HR or management, but in a peer-led team, this falls on everyone. We made a collective decision that we would all prioritise psychological safety by addressing issues as soon as they arise.

Relationships in our context go beyond professional interactions. Each team member brings their own lived experiences, often rooted in personal trauma or mental health challenges. This can sometimes create a complex interplay of emotions within the team, making it even more essential to prioritise relationships with an intentional focus on openness and understanding.

We have a clear expectation that if something feels uncomfortable or unclear, it should be brought up without delay or judgment. This does not mean we avoid discomfort; in fact, we invite difficult conversations, understanding that only by addressing tensions and uncertainties early can we maintain a safe and functional environment. The key to this is communication and the commitment to uphold our psychological safety as a shared responsibility.

This approach can sometimes be daunting. It is easy to put off difficult conversations or avoid conflict altogether, but we understand that delaying can cause tension to build in unhealthy ways. In our team, acknowledging and addressing discomfort upfront is critical for maintaining the health of our working relationships.

'No Such Thing as Too Much Information'

Another foundational belief in our team is that there is no such thing as '*too much information*'. Lived experience and peer staff often face complex personal and professional challenges that may require more communication than typically expected in a traditional work environment. We encourage our team to ask questions freely, voice their fears without hesitation, and share their thoughts without the fear of judgment or ridicule.

This is a radical shift for many who have come from workplaces where curiosity or vulnerability was seen as a weakness, or where raising personal concerns was discouraged. Here, we view these expressions as strengths. By providing a safe space for open communication, we have created an environment where people feel comfortable enough to share their anxieties, thoughts, and ideas without fear of being dismissed or invalidated. This also means that if someone feels unsure or lost, we treat their questions and concerns as valid and deserving of thoughtful attention.

This ethos invites transparency. There is no stigma attached to '*over-sharing*' or worrying about saying too much. For example, if someone needs more information on a task or seeks clarification about a decision, it is not seen as incompetence or inconvenience. Instead, it is an opportunity to build clarity and trust. By embedding this principle into our team culture, we reduce anxiety and increase the psychological safety needed for individuals to feel comfortable being their authentic selves.

Approachability and Unconditional Positive Regard

In our team, approachability is not just a personal quality – it is a shared responsibility. Every member is expected to make themselves available to listen to others, and we consciously practice unconditional positive regard for each other. This psychological term, coined by Carl Rogers, means accepting and supporting a person no matter what they are experiencing, without judgment. In a work context, it translates to making space for people's concerns and experiences, even when they are difficult to hear or understand.

The privilege of supporting others in our team is something we acknowledge often. The simple act of listening – really listening – is perhaps one of the most under-appreciated managerial tools. We believe that being available for others, without rushing to a solution or offering unasked-for advice, is critical to supporting our team's mental health and cohesion.

This requires us to constantly check in with our biases and assumptions. Are we really listening, or are we waiting for our turn to speak? Do we assume we know what the other person needs, or are we asking them directly? By ensuring that approachability is central to our ethos, we collectively create a workspace where no one feels isolated in their struggles, and everyone feels respected and heard.

Validation and Recognition

Peer staff often come from backgrounds where their experiences have been invalidated – whether by family, society, or even earlier workplaces. In our team, validation and recognition are not just nice-to-haves; they are essential practices. When someone shares their experiences, no matter how unusual or difficult they may seem, our first response is to validate. This does not mean we agree with every perspective or experience, but it does mean we acknowledge that every person's feelings are real and worthy of recognition. We strive to meet each person where they are, rather than trying to shift their perspective to meet our own. Recognition, then, is about seeing the person behind the struggle, acknowledging their contributions, and celebrating their strengths, even in moments of vulnerability.

The importance of validation extends beyond individual interactions – it is also about recognising the structural and systemic factors that shape our experiences. In a team composed of people with lived experience, it is crucial to be aware of how societal labels, discrimination, and marginalisation impact mental health. We work actively to acknowledge these dynamics rather than sweep them under the rug.

For example, if a staff member is struggling because of a past trauma that has been triggered by a particular task or interaction, we do not simply push for resilience. We validate their feelings, discuss accommodations, and recognise that these responses are part of the person's lived reality. This process ensures that the team member feels seen, heard, and respected, which is vital to fostering a trusting and secure working environment.

Managers: Flexible Thinking and Role Modelling

A final principle that underscores our team ethos is the expectation that managers model flexible thinking and problem-solving. In many ways, this stems from a reaction to past negative experiences with managers who were rigid in their approach, particularly when it came to supporting lived experience staff.

A peer-led team often includes individuals who process information and stress differently, and as a manager, it is my responsibility to guide the team in a way that respects these differences. I have learned that traditional solutions do not always work, and instead, I need to take a holistic and adaptive approach to challenges.

This involves modelling the behaviour I want to see in my team – being open about my own neurodivergence, discussing the ways I adapt to different situations, and showing how flexible thinking can lead to creative solutions. By doing this, I create a culture where difference is not just tolerated but valued.

In practice, this might look like allowing for diverse types of communication (written versus verbal), adjusting work environments to suit individual sensory needs, or providing flexibility in how tasks are completed. This approach fosters inclusivity and creates a workspace where everyone feels empowered to contribute in a way that works for them.

The Value of Lived Experience

Beyond these guiding principles, what makes managing a peer-led team particularly unique is the value that each person's lived experience brings to the service. Staff with lived experience often serve as barometers for the emotional and cultural health of the team and the broader organisation. Their ability to pinpoint discord, understand complex emotional presentations, and recognise the subtle shifts in language and behaviour are invaluable.

Peer staff are uniquely equipped to notice cultural or interpersonal issues that others might miss. They have a heightened sensitivity to power dynamics and the use of language, which can make them particularly adept at noticing when the tone of a conversation or the culture of a workplace is beginning to shift in unhealthy ways. Their insights are essential to supporting the mental health and well-being of the entire team.

Equally, lived experience staff understand the power of vulnerability. What might appear as nonsensical or overly emotional reactions to some can be re contextualised and understood through the lens of personal trauma and systemic marginalisation. In this way, the team does not just respond to distress – they engage with it thoughtfully and compassionately, seeing it as an opportunity for growth and learning.

Leadership without Ego

Perhaps the most important lesson I have learned in managing this team is the need to lead without ego. It is easy to fall into the trap of thinking that as a manager, I need to have all the answers or control every aspect of the team's functioning; in reality, the strength of our team lies in its collective knowledge and the diversity of perspectives each member brings.

As a manager, my role is to facilitate, not dictate. I need to be comfortable with uncertainty, open to learning from my team, and willing to engage in difficult conversations. This requires an ego-free approach where the primary goal is not personal success or validation, but the overall well-being and success of the team. This type of leadership also requires an awareness of power dynamics. As someone in a position of authority, I need to be mindful of how my words, actions, and decisions impact the team. This is particularly important when managing staff who may have experienced power imbalances in previous jobs or in their personal lives. By taking a reflective approach to leadership and actively seeking feedback, I strive to create a workspace where power is shared, and voices are equal.

A Holistic Approach to Team Management

Managing a peer-led team requires more than just traditional management skills. It involves creating a culture of safety, openness, and flexibility where each person feels respected and validated through actively co-creating, with all colleagues, a fundamentally inclusive workplace ethos.

Stepping into the role of managing a peer team has been one of the most transformative experiences of my professional and personal life. When I first took on this responsibility, I anticipated challenges primarily from a logistical or procedural place, as many managers would. What I encountered was an entirely new way of approaching leadership and human connection. Managing peer teams has demanded that I evolve as a person as much as I evolve my professional skills. I realised that traditional managerial mindsets of needing to be able to answer every question of provide solutions to every situation would not work here, and that I needed to shift my mindset significantly to be able to sit with uncertainty and vulnerability. I would not have associated vulnerability with leadership prior to these experiences, perhaps as a weakness or capability issue – instead, my peer teams taught me about emotional intelligence and connection. I am full of wonderful stories, all share a common thread of truly appreciating the diversity present in our team and out-of-the-box thinking that is innovative, supportive and visionary when we as leaders step back from managing and start facilitating.

Notes

1 Capturing Chapters 2–5 of this text.
2 Please note: In this chapter the terms '*lived experience*' and '*experiential knowledge*' will be used interchangeably.
3 See Chapter 3 for more details.
4 From the moment a person experiences a traumatic life event which is exacerbated by compounding factors (Norton and Cullen, 2024).
5 Role of either a service user or as a family member/carer/supporter.
6 Some of which are noted in Chapter 5.
7 A policy within the Department of Health, charged with the restructuring and transformation of the Irish health services
8 See Chapter 7 and Chapter 8 for more details on informality.
9 See Chapter 7.
10 See Chapter 4 for further details.
11 Multi-Disciplinary Team.
12 Someone with lived experience who sits on the Executive Management Team within RHAs. They are individuals with lived experience who possess a role in management.
13 Name of Irish Mental Health Services.

References

Ajjawi, R., Bearman, M., Luong, V., O'Brien, B.C. & Varpio, L. (2024) Researching lived experience in health professional education. *Medical Education* 58(9), 1049–1057. https://doi.org/10.1111/medu.15361
ANAD. (2023) Inclusive Eating Disorder Care. (Internet) Available at: https://anad.org/wp-content/uploads/2023/07/ANAD_Inclusive_Care_Guide_3.15.23.pdf, (Accessed 02nd June 2025).
Archard, P.J., O'Reilly, M., Spilsbury, T., Ali, A., Kulik, L. & Solanki, P. (2023) Informality, advocacy and the sharing of lived experience in peer support work. *Irish Journal of Psychological Medicine*. https://doi.org/10.1017/ipm.2023.8

Australian Government National Mental Health Commission (2023) *National Lived Experience (Peer) Workforce Development Guidelines: Lived Experience Workforce Development in Mental Health: A Planning Resource for Primary Health Networks* (Internet). Available at: www.mentalhealthcommission.gov.au/sites/default/files/2024-03/lived-experience-workforce-development-in-mental-health_0.pdf (Accessed 31 December 2024).

Bailie, A.H. (2015) *'From the Same Mad Planet': A Grounded Theory Study of Service User Accounts of the Relationship that develops within Professional Peer Support Work.* Ph.D Dissertation (Published), University of Nottingham, United Kingdom.

Brown, L.D., Vasquez, D., Wolf, J., Robison, J., Hartigan, L. & Hollman, R. (2024) Supporting peer support workers and their supervisors: Cluster-randomized trial evaluating a system-level intervention. *Psychiatric Services* 75(6), 514–520. https://doi.org/10.1176/appi.ps.20230112

Bureau of Justice Assistance (2022) *Bureau of Justice Assistance Comprehensive Opioid, Stimulant, and Substance Abuse Program (COSSAP) Effective Integration Toolkit: Supporting and Managing Peer Specialists: Supervision of Peer Recovery Support Services* (Internet). Available at: https://bja.ojp.gov/program/cossup/about (Accessed 02 January 2025).

Byrne, L. & Roennfeldt, H. (2024) A model of understanding lived expertise to support effective recruitment of peer roles. *Administration and Policy in Mental Health and Mental Health Services Research.* https://doi.org/10.1007/s10488-024-01424-9

Byrne, L. & Wykes, T. (2020) A role for lived experience mental health leadership in the age of Covid-19. *Journal of Mental Health* 29(3), 243–246. https://doi.org/10.1080/09638237.2020.1766002

Carswell, C., Brown, J.V.E., Lister, J., Ajjam, R.A., Alderson, S.L., Balogun-Katung, A., Bellass, S., Double, K., Gilbody, S., Hewitt, C.E., Holt, R.I.G., Jacobs, R., Kellar, I., Peckmam, E., Shiers, D., Taylor, J., Siddiqi, N. & Coventry, P. on Behalf of the DIAMONDS Research Team (2022) The lived experience of severe mental illness and long-term conditions: A qualitative exploration of service user, carer, and healthcare professional perspectives on self-managing co-existing mental and physical conditions. *BMC Psychiatry* 22, 479. https://doi.org/10.1186/s12888-022-04117-5

Castles, C., Stewart, V., Slattery, M., Bradshaw, N. & Roennfeldt, H. (2023) Supervision of the mental health lived experience workforce in Australia: A scoping review. *International Journal of Mental Health Nursing* 32(6), 1654–1671. https://doi.org/10.1111/inm.13207

Change Mental Health (n.d.) *"Shared Experiences, Shared strengths": The Power of Peer Support* (Internet). Available at: https://changemh.org/insight/shared-experiences-shared-strength-the-power-of-peer-support/#:~:text=shared%20experiences%20and%20mutual%20support,similar%20struggles%20can%20be%20comforting (Accessed 03 January 2025).

Colori, S. (2021) Dynamics of sharing lived experience. *Schizophrenia Bulletin* 48(4), 726–727. https://doi.org/10.1093/schbul/sbab076

Cooeyate, N.J., Maviglia, M. & Hume, D. (2024) The supervision gap in peer support workforce: Implications for developing effective peer support programs in native American communities. *Journal of Psychology and Clinical Psychiatry* 15(4), 211–217. https://doi.org/10.15406/jpcpy.2024.15.00783

Davey, C.G. (2022) Lived experience and the work we do. *Australian and New Zealand Journal of Psychiatry* 57(1), 5–6. https://doi.org/10.1177/00048674221144890

Dumez, V. & L'Esperance, A. (2024) Beyond experiential knowledge: A classification of patient knowledge. *Social Theory and Health* 22, 173–186. https://doi.org/10.1057/s41 285-024-00208-3

Eronen, E. (2019) Experiences of sharing, learning and caring: Peer support in a Finnish group of mothers. *Health and Social Care in the Community* 28(2), 576–583. https://doi. org/10.1111/hsc.12890

Foglesong, D., Knowles, K., Cronise, R., Wolf, J. & Edwards, J.P. (2021) National practice guidelines for peer support specialists and supervisors. *Psychiatric Services* 73(2), 215–219. https://doi.org/10.1176/appi.ps.202000901

Forbes, J. & Pratt, C.W. (2019) Can non-peer supervisors effectively supervise peer support workers? *American Journal of Psychiatric Rehabilitation* 22(3-4), 201–209. https://muse. jhu.edu/article/797609

Global Mental Health Peer Network (n.d.) *Unapologetically Experts by Experience.* (Internet) Available at: www.gmhpn.org/uploads/1/2/0/2/120276896/gmhpn_charter.pdf (Accessed 30 December 2024).

Glynn, C. (2023) *The Battle of the Peer* (Internet). Available at: https://madinireland.com/ 2023/05/the-battle-of-the-peer/ (Accessed 03 January 2025).

Goulding, R., O'Donovan, A., Drakos, K., Pierce, S., Kenny, N., Mc Dermott, S., O'Mahony, J., Venditti, V., Taylor, A., Gorman, E., Hawkins, A. & O'Malley, M. (2024) *An Exploration of the Meaning of Lived Experience and Its Application in Healthcare: A Concept Analysis and Scoping Literature Review.* University of Cork, Cork.

Gruhl, K.L.R., LaCarte, S. & Calixte, S. (2015) Authentic peer support work: Challenges and opportunities for an evolving occupation. *Journal of Mental Health.* http://dx.doi.org/ 10.3109/09638237.2015.1057322

Guarino, N., Oberle, D. & Staab, S. (2009) What is an ontology. In *Handbook on Ontologies* (Staab, S. & Studer, R. eds.). Springer, Berlin, pp. 1–17.

Hawke, L.D., Sheikhan, N.Y., Jones, N., Slade, M., Soklaridis, S., Wells, S. & Castle, D. (2022) Embedding lived experience into mental health academic research organizations: Critical reflections. *Health Expectations* 25(5), 2299–2305. https://doi.org/10.1111/ hex.13586

Health Service Executive (n.d.) *Toolkit to Support Peer Support Workers Working in the Health Service Executive* (Internet). Available at: www.hse.ie/eng/services/list/4/mental-health-services/mentalhealthengagement/peer-support-workers-toolkit.pdf (Accessed 02 January 2024).

Health Service Executive (2023) *Strategic Plan 2023–2026: Engaged in Recovery* (Internet). Available at: www.hse.ie/eng/services/list/4/mental-health-services/mental-health-eng agement-and-recovery/mher-strategic-plan-engaged-in-recovery.pdf (Accessed 30 December 2024).

Health Service Executive (2024a) *A National Framework for Recovery in Mental Health 2024–2028* (Internet). Available at: www.hse.ie/eng/services/list/4/mental-health-servi ces/mental-health-engagement-and-recovery/resources-information-and-publications/ a-national-framework-for-recovery-in-mental-health.pdf (Accessed 30 December 2024).

Health Service Executive (2024b) *Mental Health Engagement Framework 2024–2028* (Internet). Available at: www.hse.ie/eng/services/list/4/mental-health-services/mental-health-engagement-and-recovery/mental-health-engagement-framework-2024-2028.pdf (Accessed 30 December 2024).

Hunt, E. & Byrne, M. (2019) *Peer Support Workers in Mental Health Services: A Report on the Impact of Peer Support Workers in Mental Health Services* (Internet). Available at: www.lenus.ie/bitstream/handle/10147/635104/peer-support-workers-in-mental-health-services.pdf?sequence=1&isAllowed=y (Accessed 02 January 2025).

Hyde, B. (2017) *The Lived Experience of Acute Mental Health Inpatient Care: What's Recovery Got to Do With It?* Doctor of Social Work Dissertation, Charles Sturt University, Bathurst, Australia.

Kennedy, H. & Mead, S. (2019) Narrative practice and intentional peer support: A conversation between Hamilton Kennedy and Shery Mead. *The International Journal of Narrative Therapy and Community Work* 4, 50–55.

Kirkegaard, S. (2022) Experiential knowledge in mental health services: Analysing the enactment of expertise in peer support. *Sociology of Health and Illness* 44(2), 508–524. https://doi.org/10.1111/1467-9566.13438

Kivunja, C. & Kuyini, A.B. (2017) Understanding and applying research paradigms in educational contexts. *International Journal of Higher Education* 6(5), 26–41. https://doi.org/10.5430/ijhe.v6n5p26

Kumar, A., Azevedo, K.J., Factor, A., Hailu, E., Ramirez, J., Lindley, S.E. & Jain, S. (2019) Peer support in an outpatient program for veterans with posttraumatic stress disorder: Translating participant experiences into a recovery model. *Psychological Services* 16(3), 415–424. https://doi.org/10.1037/ser0000269

Lessard, E., O'Brien, N., Panaite, A.-C., Leclaire, M., Castonguay, G., Rouly, G. & Boivin, A. (2024) Can you be a peer if you don't share the same health or social condition? A qualitative study on peer integration in a primary care setting. *BMC Primary Care* 25, 298. https://doi.org/10.1186/s12875-024-02548-5

Lived Experience Workforce Program (2019) *Mental Health Peer Supervision Framework* (Internet). Available at: https://mhcsa.org.au/wp-content/uploads/2021/08/FINAL-LEWP-Peer-Supervision-Framework-111219.pdf (Accessed 02 January 2025).

Mahon, D. & Norton, M.J. (2024) The supervision of peers. In *Peer Support Work: Practice, Training and Implementation* (Mahon, D. ed.). Emerald Publishing Limited, Leeds, pp. 105–114.

Marshall, P., Babrook, J., Collins, G., Foster, S., Glossop, Z., Inkster, C., Jebb, P., Johnston, R., Jones, S.H., Khan, H., Lodge, C., Machin, K., Michalak, E., Powell, S., Russell, S., Rycroft-Malone, J., Slade, M., Whittaker, L. & Lobban, F. (2024) Designing a library of lived experience for mental health: Integrated realist synthesis and experience-based co-design study in UK mental health services. *BMJ Open* 14, e081188. https://doi.org/10.1136/bmjopen-2023-081188

Montague-Cardoso, K., Sunkel, C. & Burgess, R.A. (2024) PLOS Mental Health: Elevating the voices of lived experience to combat structural barriers and improve mental health globally. *PLOS Mental Health* 1(1), e0000053. https://doi.org/10.1371/journal.pmen.0000053

Morison, T. (2005) *Staff Supervision in Social Care*. Pavilion Publishing, Hove.

Mullineaux, L.M. (2017) *Service User Experiences of Peer Support in an Adult Community Mental Health Service: An Interpretative Phenomenological Analysis*. Ph.D Dissertation (Published), University of East Anglia, United Kingdom.

National Suicide Research Foundation (2024) *Lived Experience* (Internet). Available at: www.nsrf.ie/about-us/patient-and-public-involvement-and-engagement-ppie/#:~:text=Lived%20Experience%20(LE)%20are%20the,such%20experiences%20do%20not%20have (Accessed 30 December 2024).

Norton, M.J. (2022) More than just a health care assistant: Peer support working within rehabilitation and recovery mental health services. *Irish Journal of Psychological Medicine.* https://doi.org/10.1017/ipm.2022.32

Norton, M.J. (2023) Peer support working: A question of ontology and epistemology? *International Journal of Mental Health Systems* 17, 1. https://doi.org/10.1186/s13 033-023-00570-1

Norton, M.J. (2024) Peer work in mental health services. In *Peer Support Work: Practice Training and Implementation* (Mahon, D. ed.). Emerald Publishing Limited, Leeds, pp. 9–23.

Norton, M.J. & Cullen, O.J. (2024) Fusing experiences, reflexive thematic analysis. In *Different Diagnoses, Similar Experiences: Narratives of Mental Health, Addiction Recovery and Dual Diagnosis* (Norton, M.J. & Cullen, O.J. eds.). Emerald Publishing Limited, Leeds, pp. 177–206.

Norton, M.J., Griffin, M., Collins, M., Clark, M. & Browne, E. (2023) Using autoethnography to reflect on peer support supervision in an Irish context. *Journal of Practice Teaching and Learning* 20(1–2). https://doi.org/10.1921/jpts.v21i2.2079

Office of Mental Health Engagement and Recovery (2023) *Peer Support Epistemological Position Working Group.* Office of Mental Health Engagement and Recovery.

Owen, D., Watson, E. & Repper, J. (n.d.) *The Role of Lived Experience within Health and Social Care Systems* (Internet). Available at: https://static1.squarespace.com/static/65e87 3c27971d37984653be0/t/66bb960ec5f023459dd35bf4/1723569686714/Imroc+Brief ing+Paper+26.pdf (Accessed 30 December 2024).

Parr, S. (2023) 'Navigating' the value of lived experience in support work with multiply disadvantaged adults. *Journal of Social Policy* 52(4), 782–799. https://doi.org/10.1017/ S0047279421000921

Parsell, C., Kuskoff, E. & Constantine, S. (2024) What is the scope and contribution of lived experience in social work? A scoping review. *The British Journal of Social Work* 54(8), 3429–3448. https://doi.org/10.1093/bjsw/bcae106

Penney, D. (2018) *Who Gets to Define "Peer Support?"* (Internet). Available at: www.madin america.com/2018/02/who-gets-to-define-peer-support/ (Accessed 03 January 2025).

Plante, A. (2024) *Preserving the Heart of Peer Support: The 8 Interrelated Challenges* (Internet). Available at: www.thenationalcouncil.org/peer-support-8-interrelated-challen ges/ (Accessed 04 January 2025).

Reeves, V., Loughhead, M., Teague, C., Halpin, M.A. & Procter, N. (2024) Lived experience allyship in mental health services: Recommendations for improved uptake of allyship roles in support of peer workforce. *International Journal of Mental Health Nursing* 33(5), 1591–1601. https://doi.org/10.1111/inm.13322

Repper, J., Aldridge, B., Gilfoyle, S., Gillard, S., Perkins, R. & Rennison, J. (2013) *Peer Support Workers: A Practical Guide to Implementation* (Internet). Available at: https:// static1.squarespace.com/static/65e873c27971d37984653be0/t/668ce1d012bd721c16847 151/1720508881816/7-Peer-Support-Workers-a-practical-guide-to-implementation.pdf (Accessed 04 January 2025).

Ridley, S., Hodgson, D., Netto, J., Martin, R. & Mahboub, L. (2024) Learning about mental health lived experience in social work education. *Australian Social Work* 1–13. https:// doi.org/10.1080/0312407X.2024.2389944

Robertson, S., Leigh-Phippard, H., Robertson, D., Thomson, A., Casey, J. & Walsh, L.J. (2024) What supports the emotional well-being of peer workers in an NHS mental health service? *Mental Health and Social Inclusion.* https://doi.org/10.1108/MHSI-02-2024-0023

Sartor, C. (2023) Mental health and lived experiences: The value of lived experience expertise in global mental health. *Cambridge Prisms: Global Mental Health* 10(e38), 1–5. https://doi.org/10.1108/MHSI-02-2024-0023

Simmons, M.B., Cartner, S., MacDonald, R., Whitson, S., Bailey, A. & Brown, E. (2023) The effectiveness of peer support from a person with lived experience of mental health challenges for young people with anxiety and depression: A systematic review. *BMC Psychiatry* 23, 194. https://doi.org/10.1186/s12888-023-04578-2

Slaintecare (2017) *Committee on the Future of Healthcare: Slaintecare Report* (Internet). Available at: https://data.oireachtas.ie/ie/oireachtas/committee/dail/32/committee_on_t he_future_of_healthcare/reports/2017/2017-05-30_slaintecare-report_en.pdf (Accessed 02 January 2025).

Speyer, H., Lysaker, J.T. & Rose, D. (2024) Learning how to learn together: Integrating lived experience into mental health care. *Psychiatric Services.* https://doi.org/10.1176/appi.ps.20230607

Stichbury, J. (2017) *What Is Ontology? The Simplest Ontology Definition You'll Find ... or Your Money Back** (Internet). Available at: https://medium.com/vaticle/what-is-an-ontol ogy-c5baac4a2f6c (Accessed 31 December 2024).

Sunkel, C. & Sartor, C. (2022) Perspectives: Involving persons with lived experience of mental health conditions in service delivery, development and leadership. *BJPsych Bulletin* 46(3), 160–164. https://doi.org/10.1192/bjb.2021.51

Thoits, P.A. (2021) Successful supportive encounters from the peer supporter's perspective: Do status similarities to support recipients matter? *Journal of Community Psychology* 50(3), 1376–1394. https://doi.org/10.1002/jcop.22722

Thomson, G. & Balaam, M.-C. (2020) Sharing and modifying stories in neonatal peer support: An international mixed-method study. *Scandinavian Journal of Caring Sciences* 35(3), 805–812. https://doi.org/10.1111/scs.12895

Truong, C., Gallo, J., Roter, D. & Joo, J. (2019) The role of self-disclosure by peer mentors: Using personal narratives in depression care. *Patient Education and Counseling* 102(7), 1273–1279. https://doi.org/10.1016/j.pec.2019.02.006

Uren, E.-J. & Inder, M.L. (2021) Redefining help through peer support. *Journal of Psychiatric and Mental Health Nursing* 29(3), 390–394. https://doi.org/10.1111/jpm.12807

Wall, A., Lovheden, T., Landgren, K. & Stjernsward, S. (2022) Experiences and challenges in the role as peer support worker in a Swedish mental health context – An interview study. *Issues in Mental Health Nursing* 43(4), 344–355. https://doi.org/10.1080/01612 840.2021.1978596

Watson, E., Bowyer, D., Cooper, S., Dodd, Z., Manning, E., Morgan, G., Owen, D., Repper, J., Repper, P. & Szmit, D. (2024) *Supervision of Peer Workers* (Internet). Available at: https://static1.squarespace.com/static/65e873c27971d37984653be0/t/66b3443087061 57585716563/1723024432598/ImROC+Briefing+Paper+25+%283%29.pdf (Accessed 02 January 2025).

World Health Organization (2019) *One-to-One Peer Support by and for People with Lived Experience: WHO QualityRights Guidance Module* (Internet). Available at: https://iris.who.int/bitstream/handle/10665/329591/9789241516785-eng.pdf (Accessed 30 December 2024).

Ylonen, M. & Aven, T. (2023) A framework for understanding risk based on the concepts of ontology and epistemology. *Journal of Risk Research* 26(6), 581–593. https://doi.org/10.1080/13669877.2023.2194892

Appendix: Sample Senior Peer Support Worker Job Specifications

Job Title and Grade	Peer Support Worker, Senior (Grade Code)
Campaign Reference	
Closing Date	
Proposed Interview Date (s)	
Location of Post	
Informal Enquiries	
Details of Service	
Reporting Relationship	.
Purpose of the Post	
Principal Duties and Responsibilities	*Under the direction of the nominated line manager the Senior Peer Support Worker will:* **Professional/Admin** • Arrange and manage referral processes from teams for peer support. • Arrange and coordinate group peer support sessions as they pertain to the recovery of service users. • Work within the service and wider HSE as required to promote and develop the concept of peer support working. • Contribute, as appropriate, from a recovery perspective to the assessment, planning, implementation and review of individual care plans with the multi-disciplinary team. • Arrange coordinate and deliver training in relation to peer support. • Be aware of the competencies required for HSE Peer Support Workers. • Maintain all written records as per HSE policies. • Have a working knowledge of Mental Health Commission standards as they apply to the role. • Maintain professional standards with regard to service user and data confidentiality. • Follow up on individual issues that arise during supervision as appropriate and agreed with the supervisee. • Record and translate into themes all issues coming up during supervision to support the strategic development of peer support and recovery within services.

(Continued)

Job Title and Grade	Peer Support Worker, Senior (Grade Code)
	• Model the key principles of recovery in their work. • Demonstrate pro-active commitment to all communications with internal and external stakeholders • Keep up-to-date with organisational developments within the Irish Health Service. • Work in accordance with the principles and values of recovery as described in the *Recovery Policy Name.* **Customer Service/Service Delivery** • Ensure that service users are treated with dignity and respect. • Support the person using our services and be aware of their rights within the service and the supports available to access these. • Be aware of the Human Rights legislation in relation to the requirements of this post. • Promote equality of opportunity and good relations as outlined in the *organisation's* equality policy • Facilitate opportunities for people using our services to direct their own recovery, based on the recovery principles. • Promote and support independent living for people using our services, signposting to their local community and developing connections with family, friends and significant others where appropriate. • Act on feedback from service users and report the same to the Line Manager. **Human Resources/Supervision of Staff** • Provide supervision at a group and individual level to Peer Support Workers and other staff with lived experience as required working in their service area. • Use a strengths-based approach to consistently give recognition and praise for competency development and successful outputs/outcomes with service users. • Have the capacity to give and receive feedback, creating support and trust. • Encourage Peer Support Workers to discuss openly any challenges or difficulties that they have or are experiencing within their team and with service users.

Job Title and Grade	Peer Support Worker, Senior (Grade Code)
	• Provide role clarity to Peer Support Workers of the task required, and about what is appropriate to self-disclose. • Use supervision as a medium to identify, discuss and process situations where there is confusion about the Peer Support Worker role. • Promotes and monitors the self-care and wellness of the Peer Support Worker. • Model good self-care and health maintenance, including a system of support. • Work in partnership with Peer Support Workers in the development of a meaningful work plan for peer support work. • Provide signposting to ongoing training and support Peer Support Workers to access ongoing education/training/coaching opportunities. • Afford opportunities for participation and training to all staff equally, including Peer Support Workers. • Assists Peer Support Workers in understanding the organisation's policies and procedures to safeguard and maintain the safety and health of the Peer Support Worker. • Assists Peer Support Workers to access community health care resource directories and facilitate the sharing of community resource information within the team. • Be aware of ethical standards for all staff and boundary issues common with Peer Support Workers and also those specific to their profession. • Be accessible, maintain regular supervision appointments and provide consistent availability for crisis support. • Practices good time management and respects the supervision contract, keeping supervision appointments and being present and accessible to the Peer Support Worker. • Supervise the delivery of recovery and peer-based work remotely as stipulated under the Peer Support Distance Working guidance document published by the HSE Mental Health Services in 2020.

(Continued)

Job Title and Grade	Peer Support Worker, Senior (Grade Code)
	• Support the Peer Support Worker in understanding their rights and entitlements as an employee of the HSE mental health services. • Support Peer Support Workers to plan and risk-assess work to be carried out without close or direct supervision, in line with the local Lone Worker Policy and Procedures. **Health and Safety** • Promote a safe working environment in accordance with Health and Safety legislation. • Be aware of and implement agreed policies, procedures and safe professional practice by adhering to relevant legislation, regulations and standards. • Actively participate in risk management issues, identify risks and take responsibility for appropriate action. • Document appropriately and report any adverse incidents, near misses, hazards and accidents in accordance with organisational guidelines. • Have a working knowledge of the Health Information and Quality Authority (HIQA) Standards as they apply to the role, for example Standards for Healthcare, National Standards for the Prevention and Control of Healthcare Associated Infections and Hygiene Standards and comply with associated protocols for implementing and maintaining these standards as appropriate to the role. • Support, promote and actively participate in sustainable energy, water and waste initiatives to create a more sustainable, low-carbon and efficient health service. **Education and Training** • Attend induction and mandatory in-service education relevant to the role. • Participate in the induction of new staff as directed. • Participate in Performance Achievement in conjunction with the line manager. • Participate in team-based development, education, training and learning.

Job Title and Grade	Peer Support Worker, Senior (Grade Code)

Eligibility Criteria Qualifications and/or Experience	**Candidates must have by the closing date for receipt of applications for this post:**
	
	1. **Professional Qualifications, Experience etc.**
	  (a) Be working as a Peer Support Worker for a period of no less than 3 years.
	    And
	  (b) Hold a certificate in peer support working in mental health.
	    And
	  (c) Have previous experience of supervising staff
	2. **Health**
	  A candidate for and any person holding the office must be fully competent and capable of undertaking the duties attached to the office and be in a state of health such as would indicate a reasonable prospect of ability to render regular and efficient service.
	3. **Character**
	  Each candidate for and any person holding the office must be of good character ....

Post Specific Requirements	• Be willing to undergo specific training in clinical supervision • Demonstrate depth and breadth of experience working with Peer Support Worker colleagues and multi-disciplinary team members with which such individuals are likely to engage over the course of their work. • Experience in supporting and promoting the implementation of self-care frameworks and approaches, as relevant to the role. • Demonstrate the ability to organise and prioritise tasks as it relates to the management of one's own workload and that of their Peer Support Worker colleagues in which they supervise.
Other Requirements	• Access to appropriate personal transport is a necessary requirement to carry out the duties and responsibilities of this post. • Ability to work in a flexible way, informed by line management and their junior colleagues' needs.

(Continued)

Job Title and Grade	Peer Support Worker, Senior (Grade Code)
Skills, Competencies and/or Knowledge	Candidates must demonstrate the following: **Professional Knowledge** • A willingness to use a strengths-based approach to consistently give recognition and praise for competency development and successful outputs/outcomes for service users. • An awareness of the competencies required for Peer Support Workers. • Knowledge of how recovery works in Mental Health Services and be aware of their service's recovery framework. • The key principles of recovery in their personal work. • Recognition of the value of the recovery capital/assets of peer support working. • An understanding of the natural support system of Peer Support Workers including family, and allies and other strengths-based approaches to support recovery. • An awareness of the importance of instilling hope, often facilitated through appropriate self-disclosure and empathy. • An understanding of the importance of lived experience and the value of peers as a bridge between traditional behavioural health institutions and the natural supports of friends, families, allies and the greater recovery community. • Knowledge and experience of self-care frameworks and approaches in the context of mental health recovery. • In-depth knowledge of the inner workings of the Mental Health Services. • Knowledge of mental health policy and procedures as it relates to peer support working. • Knowledge of employee safety mechanisms and encourage a culture of acknowledging and learning from mistakes/errors. • Knowledge of current best practices and procedures within mental health recovery, social inclusion and peer support working. • Basic knowledge of ICT.

Job Title and Grade	Peer Support Worker, Senior (Grade Code)
	Planning and Organising Skills • Organisational and time management skills so as to prioritise work based on the junior Peer Support Worker's and their own work plan needs • The ability to work to tight deadlines and operate effectively with multiple competing priorities. **Leadership and Teamwork** • Capacity to operate successfully in challenging operational environments while adhering to quality standards. • Leadership potential, the ability to manage the performance of others and support staff development • The ability to be flexible and adapt to change. • Teamwork skills including the ability to work in a multi-disciplinary team environment (i.e. in a team with other disciplines). • The capacity to operate successfully in a challenging operational environment while adhering to quality standards. • Motivation and an innovative approach to the job within a changing working environment. • The ability to work independently, in a range of settings and as appropriate. **Commitment to Providing a Quality Service** • A core belief in and passion that will support the supervisee in sustaining the delivery of high-quality service user-focused services. • Commitment to recovery-focused principles and practices within their own work and their supervisory duties. • Commitment to their continuous professional development. **Communication and Interpersonal Skills** • Effective interpersonal skills. • Effective written and verbal communication skills; including the ability to present information in a clear and concise manner. • The ability to form peer relationships with people using our services and supportive relationships with family members. • The ability to interact in a professional manner with other Mental Health staff and other key stakeholders.

(Continued)

Job Title and Grade	Peer Support Worker, Senior (Grade Code)
Campaign-Specific Selection Process Ranking/Shortlisting/ Interview	
Code of Practice	
This job description is a guide to the general range of duties assigned to the post holder. It is intended to be neither definitive nor restrictive and is subject to periodic review with the employee concerned.	

Chapter 7

Models of Peer Support Work

7.1 Introduction

In the previous chapter of this text, we explored lived experience and its knowledge set – experiential knowledge in detail. This included gaining a consensus from the literature as to the key characteristics that make up a definition for the knowledge set used, through to its philosophical positioning as well as issues pertaining to remaining authentic to lived experience and the sharing of such expertise within the clinical setting. This present chapter expands on this by discussing models as to how peer support work actually occurs in mental health service provision. This begins with Section 7.2 where a model I developed as a student will be explored. This model advocates for a mechanism of sharing lived experiences as well as re-enforcing the importance of sharing the same. Within Section 7.2, I will also tackle a commonality identified among these models of peer support working – that of discharge given the close, friend-like relationship[1] that develops as a result. However, as alluded to a moment ago, this model of peer support work does not stand in isolation. Section 7.3 will briefly review other models of peer support working applicable to a mental health context. Finally, Section 7.4 ends the chapter by summarising what has been learnt as well as touching on elements that will be addressed in the next chapter of this text. 'Section 7.2: The Stepping Model' is now presented.

7.2 The Stepping Model

Peer Support Workers have been employed in many different roles and settings (Repper et al., 2013; Gillard et al., 2022). As a result, this has led to much role conflict and indeed confusion (Jacobson et al., 2012; Kim and Kweon, 2024). To address such confusion, I, with the support of my supervisors at that time, constructed a model of peer support working in mental health through an unpublished meta-synthesis of the available literature at the time (2019/20) (Norton et al., 2020). A meta-synthesis is a type of literature review focused on synthesising primary qualitative literature in either an aggregative or interpretative approach to construct new meaning which serves to advance the field of knowledge (Sim and

DOI: 10.4324/9781032717050-10

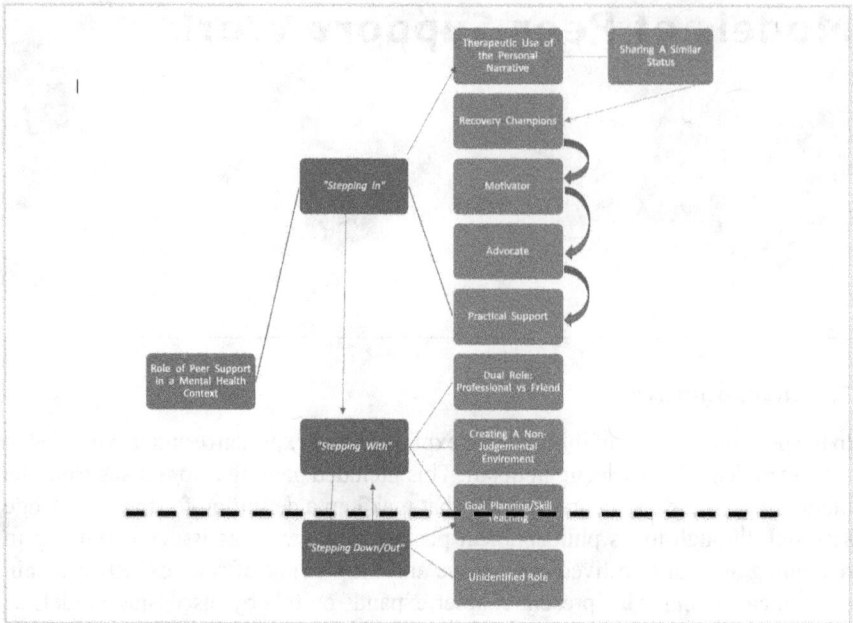

Figure 7.1 The Stepping Model.

Mengshoel, 2022; McLeod, 2024). This model of peer support working is known as '*The Stepping Model*' which is visually illustrated in Figure 7.1 and discussed in further detail.

Figure created as part of an unpublished systematic review and meta-synthesis by Norton et al. (2020).

7.2.1 'Stepping In'

'*Stepping In*' marks the first stage of '*The Stepping Model*' and represents the day of the first appointment with the service user who is to be in receipt of peer support (Norton, 2024). At the beginning of the relationship with the service user, there is a hidden hierarchy evident between both parties. This hidden hierarchy is evoked from the service user's perception of the peer as a mental health service provider. Someone who holds within them all the wisdom required to enable this individual to recover. This perception, although natural, has the potential to damage the peer relationship as peers are supposed to work on a more intimate basis than what other service providers are capable and allowed to achieve over the course of their work. As such, the aim of the peer in the first instance is to destroy any hierarchical blockades that inhibit the peer relationship to create a space known as informality (Norton, 2022). It is within this space that more candid conversations can begin that act as catalysts for recovery (Norton et al., 2023). To begin this process of tearing down the hierarchical blockades, the peer utilises their personal narrative in a therapeutic manner. As noted in the previous chapter, there is still much debate regarding what and how narratives/lived experiences can be shared. In the case of '*The Stepping Model*', based on the evidence available at that time along with my own personal experiences of providing peer support, we identified that such sharing of lived experiences occurs through the sharing of similarities and not the entire narrative.

Regardless of what mechanism is employed in the sharing of lived experiences within peer support work, the result remains the same. That is the transformation of the peer from the viewpoint of being just another service provider to that of a recovery champion. This then evokes a motivation within the service user themselves to look at their own lives and stride towards recovery. Additionally, it is documented that Peer Support Workers are not advocates for the individuals they work with (Marks et al., 2022; Norton, 2024). However, at this early stage of the peer relationship, further blockades from other providers involved in their care may be placed in front of the service user, requiring careful attention to be safely removed without damaging the relationship. Additionally, the service user may be in a very early stage of their recovery journey and as a result may not have the capacity, faculty or confidence to advocate for themselves. Only on these occasions should the peer act as a temporary advocate to remove the blockade so that informality can occur. The peer should remain in the advocate position for as little time as possible until the service user has the ability to advocate for themselves again.

Often, as is the case described by Norton (2022) in his letter to the editor, the location in which peer support work occurs can also be a factor in creating a hierarchy. For example, acute inpatient settings or hostels are manned by staff who work within the rehabilitation and recovery mental health services and so on. As a result, the peer will often engage in their work in informal surroundings like cafés, shopping centres or even through a game of Connect Four or chess. What is done and what environment surrounds the activity of peer support is not important. What is important here is how what is being done and the environment around it is reflective of informal activity. It is the placement of where peer support occurs and the activity that both parties engage in whilst practising peer support work that is the final ingredient in what creates a state of informality. This marks the end of the '*Stepping In*' phase of '*The Stepping Model*'. The timeline in creating informality may be as little as one meeting but can take several attempts, particularly if the individual concerned, like in Norton's example, is returning to a place of hierarchy after the session closes. It is at the point of creation of informality that all hierarchical blockades are eradicated and that the relationship enters the next phase of the model, labelled here as '*Stepping With*'.

7.2.2   'Stepping With'

As noted above, once a state of informality is achieved, the '*Stepping In*' phase ends and the '*Stepping With*' phase begins. Through the creation of informality, a friend-like relationship is formed. This, as noted earlier, culminates from the breakdown of hierarchical barriers so that what is left are two people, who are equal to one another and are connected through life experiences working together towards the same end goal. Again, this does not suggest that once informality is created, it stays static. In fact, informality is fluid and depending on the life situation of the individual the peer is supporting, it may be necessary to constantly construct, break down and construct informality again. As such, the peer should enter each session with a check on social, environmental and interventional factors that may influence this fluidity so that a state of informality can be maintained.

The friend-like relationship that is created as a result of informality resembles that of an actual friendship, but there are rules attached to it. This is because the peer is an employee of the services and, as such, must abide by the rules and regulations that govern the organisation in question. This usually means that the service user has access to the peer Monday to Friday, between the hours of 9 am to 5 pm. The peer cannot be in contact after that or on weekends. The service user is to pay for their own refreshments at a coffee shop, and the relationship is not everlasting. In other words, there is an endpoint to the relationship, after which all communication 'technically' ceases.[2] As such, the peer must sit within a tenuous position by occupying both a formal and informal role[3] all at one time. The advantage of informality is not only in terms of mutuality and reciprocity[4] but also in the creation of a non-judgemental environment. This non-judgemental environment along with the other components of informality allows for the recipient of peer support to take a step back and explore their own ill health and recovery journey so that they can decide for themselves what they want for their life and recovery and what steps they need to take to get to this ideal. The 'Stepping With' phase ends once the goals set out by the service user are acted upon and have reached some way towards completion.

7.2.3   'Stepping Down/Out'

As the 'Stepping With' phase ends, the 'Stepping Down/Out' begins. This phase represents the final stage of the relationship where goals are reached and completed, and the relationship with the peer begins to slow down to the point of discharge from peer services (Norton, 2024). However, at the time of writing, there remains no consensus regarding the discharge of the service user from a friend-like therapeutic relationship like that created in peer support work. In fact, there seems to be a paucity of evidence when it comes to this particular aspect of peer support working. What is known is that ending the relationship is not only difficult for the service user but also for the Peer Support Workers themselves (Watson, 2016). Spotlight on Mental Health (2012) has identified several tips that can be used in such a scenario to support the Peer Support Worker and the service user. These include:

- Reviewing goals and acknowledging achievements.
- Preparing the service user ahead of time – at least one month's prior notice.
- Letting the service user know that you are proud of them and provide examples of how they have grown since commencing peer support work.

- Evaluating their experience of the peer support service. What was helpful and what could be improved?
- Acknowledging and validating feelings of loss.
- Encouraging the service user to speak to their other supports.
- Pointing out strengths as well as the other relationships and skills they have developed.
- Letting the service user know the impact they have had on your life and that you will miss them also.
- Thanking the service user.
- Re-enforcing the fact that the goals achieved were their achievement, not yours and providing reassurance that they can continue without you.

(Spotlight on Mental Health, 2012)

You may also notice that there are two arrows between '*Stepping With*' and '*Stepping Down/Out*'. These arrows represent in a lot of ways the fluidity of the model and indeed of recovery itself. In the process of weaning the service user off the Peer Support Worker, the service user may, for a multitude of reasons, begin to become unwell again and take a step backwards in their recovery. In such a case, the peer returns to the '*Stepping With*' phase, re-establishes informality and engages in dialogue with the service user to identify what has happened, what new goals need to be set in order for the service user to live their best life and plan a timeline for the successful completion of these goals. It is at this point that the peer can move back to the '*Stepping Down/Out*' phase and slowly, at a pace that is suitable for the situation, conclude the relationship.

7.3 Other Models of Peer Support Work

There is a sparse amount of literature that examines actual models of peer support working. Instead, the literature uses the terms type and model interchangeably. An example of where this is the case is in The Housing Agency (2024) report on peer support models, where in fact they refer to types of peer support work. To the best of the author's knowledge, only one other paper, Zeng and Chung (2019), actually presented a model of peer work: '*The Stepped Model of Peer Provider Practice*' (Figure 7.2) that could be critically reviewed and applied to mental health service provision. A stepped model was chosen to showcase the non-linearity of the peer relationship and indeed the recovery journey also. As a result, the peer can move fluidly along '*The Stepped Model of Peer Provider Practice*' like a continuum. '*The Stepped Model of Peer Provider Practice*' consists of three stages: '*Creating a Safe Place*', '*Working Partnership*' and '*Stepping Out*'. These are explored further.

7.3.1 '*Creating a Safe Place*'

'*Creating a Safe Place*' is the first phase of this model of peer support work (Zeng and Chung, 2019). It involves the creation and building of trust. This begins with

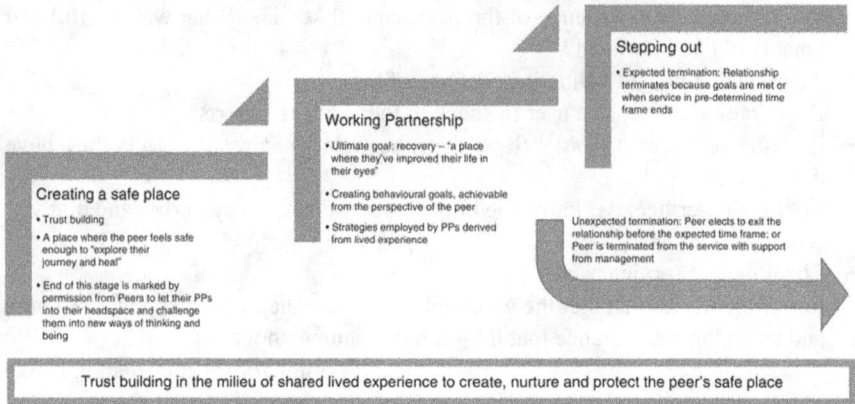

Figure 7.2 The Stepped Model of Peer Provider Practice.

meeting the service user where they are at in terms of their recovery. This often requires the peer to be present with the person in distress. Within this model, creating a safe place is achieved through two processes: making a connection and holding hope in the milieu of shared lived experiences. In creating a connection with the service user, the peer should view the individual as a person and not a set of symptoms. This is achieved by getting to know the service user and developing and intimate knowledge of who they are. Part of this is looking at the common experience of mental distress and sharing such intimate details of the peer's own lived experiences with the service user. This creates a deep connection as the peer and service user both understand what it is like to be seen as an illness and through the peer's recovery journey, become a new identity, away from that of illness. Once the creation of a safe place is confirmed, this first phase of the model is complete (Zeng and Chung, 2019).

7.3.2 'Working Partnership'

Once the safe space is created, the '*Working Partnership*' phase begins. This involves a process of goal identification and setting to help the service user towards recovery. These goals are often behavioural in nature and achievable in the eyes of the Peer Support Worker. Once a suitable goal is identified, a plan is created to support the attainment of that goal. Then the service user goes about achieving this goal and is accountable to their Peer Support Worker. The Peer Support Worker can also empower the peer through a process of role modelling, and storytelling through the use of aspects of the narrative that can instil hope and that offer a different perspective of a situation the service user is faced with or through cognitive strategies like mindfulness and cognitive behavioural therapy. However, with these strategies of empowerment – particularly the cognitive strategies – it is important to note that the Peer Support Worker conducts the same from a different knowledge base and epistemological understanding to that of other non-peer professionals that is afforded to them due to their lived experiences (Zeng and Chung, 2019; Norton, 2024a). Once all the goals in the person's plan of care are achieved, the '*Working Partnership*' phase ends.

7.3.3 'Stepping Out'

The '*Stepping Out*' phase marks the end of the relationship with the service user. According to Zeng and Chung (2019), there are two circumstances by which the peer support relationship ends. The first occurs in an expected time frame that is governed by either the attainment of the identified goals or a time frame set by the multi-disciplinary team. In this first circumstance, the Peer Support Worker is noted to intentionally prepare the service user for a life without the peer's influence. The start of this occurs at the '*Creating a Safe Place*' phase of this model. In other words, it occurs at the beginning of the relationship with the service user. The second circumstance that results in the end of the peer support relationship occurs in an unexpected time frame where the service users themselves may elect to exit the relationship, possibly because they are not finding it beneficial. Additionally, the Peer Support Workers themselves may elect to exit the relationship due to the lack of progress towards the identified goals. In most cases, the first circumstance is the one chosen, with the closure of the relationship marked by both parties becoming involved in something special like getting a cake or going paintball shooting and so on. It is at this point the '*Stepping Out*' phase concludes and the model reaches its completion.

7.4 Concluding Remarks

Peer support work, in a professional/formalised capacity, is a relatively new phenomenon within mental health service provision and represents the most recent advances in mental health discourse (Davidson et al., 2012; Tse et al., 2017). The present chapter explored two specific peer support working models – one developed through the previous work of the author and the other from Zeng and Chung (2019). Ironically, both suggest that their models are stepped in nature and illustrate the relationship from the moment it begins to the ending of the relationship. An interesting concept for future study is the exact mechanism of discharge from peer support services that ensures that the strong friend-like attachment created because of informality does not end up harming either party involved. As we now move forward to the next chapter of this text, we will explore this tenuous relationship amongst other debated factors further to analyse their ethical implications for peer support working in mental health.

Notes

1   This is touched on in this chapter in order to explain The Stepping Model but will be explored in a lot more detail in Chapter 8.
2   The word '*technically*' is added as in a lot of these situations, the peer relationship may end, but the bond forged between both individuals becomes an actual friendship once the work is completed.
3   This is explored in more depth in Chapter 8.
4   Both principles of peer support work. See Chapter 4 for more details.

References

Davidson, L., Bellamy, C., Guy, K. & Miller, R. (2012) Peer support among persons with severe mental illnesses: A review of evidence and experience. *World Psychiatry* 11(2), 123–128. https://doi.org/10.1016/j.wpsyc.2012.05.009

Gillard, S., Foster, R., White, S., Barlow, S., Bhattacharya, R., Binfield, P., Eborall, R., Faulkner, A., Gibson, S., Goldsmith, L.P., Simpson, A., Licock, M., Marks, J., Morshead, R., Patel, S., Priebe, S., Repper, J., Rinaldi, M., Ussher, M. & Worner, J. (2022) The impact of working as a peer worker in mental health services: A longitudinal mixed methods study. *BMC Psychiatry* 22, 373. https://doi.org/10.1186/s12888-022-03999-9

Jacobson, N., Trojanowski, L. & Dewa, C.S. (2012) What do peer support workers do? A job description. *BMC Health Services Research* 12, 205. https://doi.org/10.1186/1472-6963-12-205

Kim, S-Y. & Kweon, Y-R. (2024) The poetry of recovery in peer support workers with mental illness: An interpretative phenomenological analysis. *Healthcare* 12(2), 123. https://doi.org/10.3390/healthcare12020123

Marks, J., Sriskandarajah, N., Aurelio, M.M., Gillard, S., Rinaldi, M., Foster, R. & Ussher, M. (2022) Experiences of peer workers and mental health service users with a peer support intervention: Applying and critiquing a behaviour change techniques taxonomy. *Advances in Mental Health* 20(2), 91–101. https://doi.org/10.1080/18387357.2021.2012088

McLeod, S. (2024) *Metasynthesis of Qualitative Research* (Internet). Available at: https://www.simplypsychology.org/metasynthesis.html (Accessed 6 January 2025).

Norton, M.J. (2022) More than just a health care assistant: Peer support working within rehabilitation and recovery mental health services. *Irish Journal of Psychological Medicine*. https://doi.org/10.1017/ipm.2022.32

Norton, M.J. (2024a) Peer work in mental health services. In *Peer Support Work: Practice, Training and Implementation* (Mahon, D. ed.). Emerald Publishing Limited, Leeds, pp. 9–23.

Norton, M.J. (2024b) Using learned tools for experiential gain: The application of experiential knowledge to traditional service processes. *Irish Journal of Psychological Medicine*. https://doi.org/10.1017/ipm.2024.4

Norton, M.J., Archard, P. & Swords, C. (2023) The ethics of informality and dual relationships in peer support. *Psychiatric Services* 74(2), 2. https://doi.org/10.1176/appi.ps.20230291

Norton, M.J., Bergin, M. & Denieffe, S. (2020) Service user views of peer support in mental health: A systematic review and meta-synthesis. Unpublished Manuscript.

Repper, J., Aldridge, B., Gilfoyle, S., Gillard, S., Perkins, R. & Rennison, J. (2013) *Peer Support Workers: Theory and Practice* (Internet). Available at: https://recoverycontextinventory.com/images/resources/ImROC_peer_support_workers_theory_practice.pdf (Accessed 6 January 2025).

Sim, J. & Mengshoel, A.M. (2022) Metasynthesis: Issues of empirical and theoretical context. *Quality and Quantity* 57, 3339–3361. https://doi.org/10.1007/s11135-022-01502-w

Spotlight on Mental Health (2012) *Peer Support Relationships: Tips for Ending Well* (Internet). Available at: https://spotlightonmentalhealth.com/peer-support-relationships-tips-for-ending-well/ (Accessed 9 January 2025).

The Housing Agency (2024) *Peer Support Models: Examining Models both Nationally and Internationally* (Internet). Available at: www.housingagency.ie/sites/default/files/2024-12/The%20Housing%20Agency%20-%20Action%202.2.3%20a%20Peer%20Support%20Models_0.pdf (Accessed 10 January 2025).

Tse, S., Mak, W.W.S., Lo, I.W.K., Liu, L.L., Yuen, W.W.Y., Yau, S., Ho, K., Chan, S-K. & Wong, S. (2017) A one-year longitudinal qualitative study of peer support services in a non-western context: The perspectives of peer support workers, service users, and co-workers. *Psychiatry Research* 255, 27–35. https://doi.org/10.1016/j.psychres.2017.05.007

Watson, E. (2016) A day in the life of a peer support worker: ending. *Mental Health and Social Inclusion* 20(1), 17–21. https://doi.org/10.1108/MHSI-01-2016-0001

Zeng, G. & Chung, D. (2019) The stepped model of peer provision practice: Capturing the dynamics of peer support work in action. *The Journal of Mental Health Training, Education and Practice* 14(2), 106–118. https://doi.org/10.1108/JMHTEP-09-2018-0052

Chapter 8

Ethical Dilemmas in Peer Support Work

Case Study Contributor:

Karen Beveridge and Nina Eck

8.1 Introduction

In the previous chapter, we explored two specific models of peer support working in mental health. Both discussed the journey the peer and service user undertake to first build trust and then once trust is attained, to support the service user in the identification and attainment of service user-appointed goals. All of this leads to a point of discharge, where the service user learns to live a life of their own choosing in the absence of peer support input. Every aspect of this process raises practical and ethical concerns that need to be understood in detail and addressed accordingly in order for the peer support relationship to maintain its therapeutic value.

In this present chapter, such issues are explored in depth. This begins with Section 8.2 which will critically discuss the maintenance of a dual role within peer support work. This will link in with previous discussions regarding the creation of informality, but this time we will enhance such discussions by exploring the phenomena of '*ethical informality*'. Following on from this, Section 8.3 will explore the ethical dilemmas raised as a result of working in a service/location/team where one was formally a patient. Given the ethical issues documented here, the supervision of the peer yet again forms part of our discussions within Section 8.4. In particular, we will explore the process of supervision and how it should operate within peer support work to support those peers who encounter such ethical dilemmas over the course of their work. Additionally, Section 8.5 will examine peer support work training in depth and will discuss what elements should be included in the training of the peer. The chapter then concludes with a summary of what has been explored here in Section 8.6. These subsections will be supported by a series of case studies detailing the personal experiences of peers in the field dealing with these ethical dilemmas in practice.

8.2 The Maintenance of a Dual Role: Professional and Friend

As stipulated in a previous chapter,[1] the creation of the tenuous position of both professional and friend is made as a side effect of the creation of informality – a space of pure mutuality and reciprocity resulting from the destruction of all hierarchical blockades. Informality creates other ethical concerns too which are discussed

DOI: 10.4324/9781032717050-11

further in Section 8.2.1. However, for this part of the chapter, we will examine the ethical dilemma of the dual role in peer support work and how this impacts the work these practitioners do daily.

The identification of a dual role complex in peer support work was first noted by Davidson et al. (2006) when they first illustrated the same through a continuum of helping relationships (Figure 8.1). However, it was not till 2010 when Barlow and colleagues first identified the potential issues around the maintenance of the dual role. This was noted on the front line, where peers worked with individuals, but could not recognise or maintain this non-hierarchical space (Barlow et al., 2010).

Similar findings were also noted by Faulkner and Basset (2010) and Shaw et al. (2009), where Shaw and colleagues recognised the space by comparing the same to an old weighing scale where one is to remain balanced between the '*friend*' that service users are familiar with and the '*professional*' which is observed in the eyes of the services. Such balancing may take time to perfect due to an individual's past experiences and because the mechanism whereby the scales remain level differs from one service user to the next.

Indeed Boardman et al. (2015) add to this by suggesting that the boundaries imposed on the peer by the system that views them as a professional can indeed impede the practicing of the peer role to its most authentic state. For instance, most peers work only during office hours and as such cannot support service users after 5 pm on a weekday. In addition, peers cannot stay with the service user for

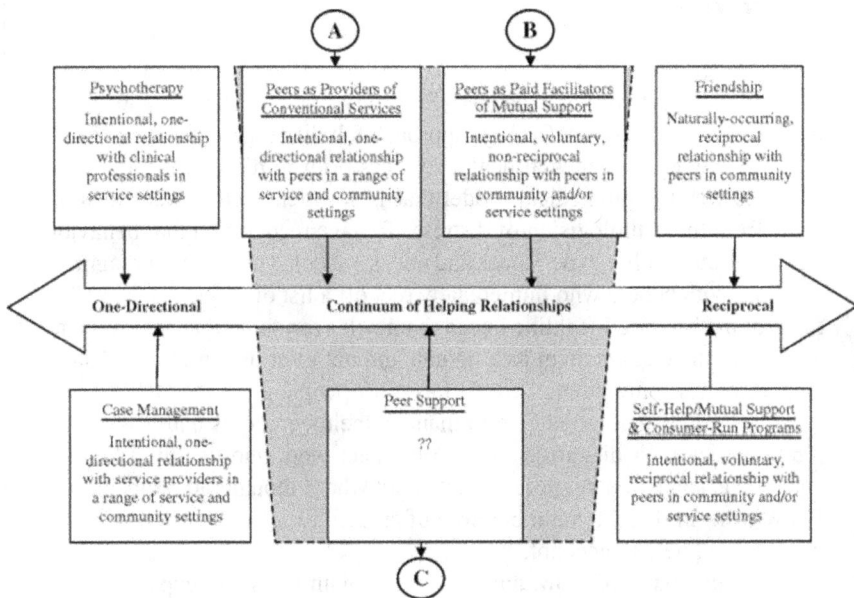

Figure 8.1 A Continuum of Helping Relationships among Adults with Serious Mental Illness.

a prolonged period of time as the system requires the peer to achieve results in a relatively short period of time. Now this is based on the lack of understanding of the essence of the peer relationship by the multi-disciplinary team as well as the organisation that the peer inherently works for.

Smedburg (2015) adds to this by suggesting that this dual role can lead in itself to a lack of role clarity, particularly towards where the peer role begins and ends. This lack of clarity in particular occurs when one transitions between the '*friend*' and '*professional*' identity (Walker and Bryant, 2013). For instance, in the maintenance of informality, a peer may meet a service user at the cinema, or at a youth club. Both of these inherently are informal locations where both parties engage in informal activity. However, when the peer writes in the clinical notes, the peer must utilise the science of peer support working to detail to other staff what mechanisms are invisibly at play within these informal settings and activities that inherit an outcome that can be noted within a care plan. In this way, role confusion can result from the transformation of informal activity to a professional document, but also when a professional reads the notes of a peer that engages in informal activity leading to queries as to whether the peer is (1) impeding on the space of other care staff and (2) if the peer is doing their actual job or just having fun. In Case Study 7, Karen further explores the intricacies of working in an in-between tenuous space as a Peer Support Worker in the UK.

Case Study 7   Working in the in between Space as a Peer Worker

Karen Beveridge

I work as a peer worker in an NHS Recovery College. The role appealed to me because the Recovery College approach felt different to what I was used to. My experience of mental health services prior to discovering Recovery Colleges was the biomedical model that is so often used. I want to move away from the pathologising of distress. To have recognition that behaviour can be because of life experiences and not as a set of symptoms for diagnosis. Working with people who immediately reel off a list of diagnosis is challenging for me because I feel like I need to unpick everything that has happened to them to understand them as a human and not a set of symptoms. That of course creates some internal conflict as most people go to the NHS to get a diagnosis and usually medicine to manage their symptoms and it is not my job to unpick their diagnosis. When I did peer work unofficially, I had less constraints and could be more honest about what I thought about the system I now work in. I felt I could be more of an activist, often labelled '*difficult*' by services I held to account.

I'm a '*professional*' now, and that comes with rules and expectations of how a professional communicates and behaves. However, doing this within the third sector or as a peer in a support group that I attended to help myself often meant being under supported, trained and supervised unless I took the initiative to learn good practice.

My own experience of the system was basically me giving up my power and surrendering to being ill, taking medication and '*doing as I was told*' in cognitive behavioural therapy (CBT) sessions. Nobody ever wanted to explore why I behaved the way I did or felt sad and numb all the time. I was told by the CBT practitioner that my life was overwhelming, I felt crushed under the weight of my responsibilities and historic trauma. I felt like I was told I wasn't trying hard enough to think positively. After all, '*if I changed the way I think it would change the way I behave*'. CBT didn't work for me, and I suspect it isn't as effective for many people who have conditions in life beyond their control. People facing economic struggles, poor housing, systematic injustice and not fitting in.

I wanted to come into the role and be the person that didn't take away their power, dignity or safety. I wanted to be the person I needed when I was experiencing distress. I feel valued in my role and don't feel like I must model wellness. The way I see it is that I'm there because of my lived experience, if I'm pretending to have it all together, I won't be relatable anyway. But, having spoken to other peers it does seem like they are expected to present as '*recovered*' rather than as someone who understands what care may look like and offer a non-oppressive option. That if they experience instability they may not be seen as professional as another worker. I feel like sometimes we are there to be rolled out to show that the system works, not to say that we are there to advocate and try to change the system that may have caused them harm.

When I talk to the humans I am asked to work with, which we refer to as learners I often hear things they are dissatisfied with. A lot of their dissatisfaction is tied with other professionals not hearing them, because of my lived experience/professional crossover I like to think I can see things from both perspectives. Firstly, as the potentially overworked tired professional who lacks the energy to listen to everything and pick out everything that they can practically do. I suspect they just hear feelings and disengage, missing opportunities to hear valuable feedback that can be used to improve services. With my experience of living this for myself I listen carefully and pick out those things that can be presented in a concise way and deliver those messages to the people who didn't hear it at the first opportunity. I also have a valuable opportunity to validate the feelings of the learner and hopefully try and make some reparations. It is possible to retain your job and acknowledge that everything isn't perfect with the organisation you are employed by. I am however vigilant to not cross the line too much as I hope for career progression. Perhaps this is why many survivors are critical of peer workers being employed by the services they feel they had to survive?

I am aware my experience is not representative of what other peers may experience; I am fortunate enough to be in a supportive team where everyone is willing to discuss lived experiences. Not that distress, grief or trauma somehow bypasses you if you are a manager and that only I must show my vulnerability as that is my job. That supportive team is also available for quality supervision, to facilitate group supervision and allow time for reflection and to learn from the lived experiences of others.

Interestingly in my research for career progression within my NHS trust it appears that my options for progression keeping my lived experience angle are limited. However, I think if I had to compromise my values, I have developed due to my lived experience, I would struggle to assimilate into a role that didn't involve my lived experience.

In Karen's case study, she has highlighted the inability, thanks to the professional side of her role to critique and advocate for a change in the way the system operates as she is afraid this would impact her own career progression. However, she has highlighted the importance of referring back to her own lived experiences to balance this role out. Section 8.2.1 will now discuss the creation and maintenance of informality – the phenomenon responsible for the creation of a dual role – and how this can lead to ethical dilemmas within the practice of peer support work.

8.2.1   The Creation of Informality

Informality was first identified by Norton (2022) where he defined it as an interpersonal, reciprocal and mutually exclusive space that is constructed by the Peer Support Worker over the course of their work. It is brought about, in part through the sharing of aspects of ones lived experiences and through the informal environments where such experiences are expressed and indeed where such interactions take place. Informality is important in peer support as it is through its creation that discussions are facilitated to (1) address the mental health challenge, but more importantly (2) what the individual wants for their recovery and indeed their life. It is through the creation of informality that a dual role is born: one of professional and one of friend. This was first identified by Davidson et al. (2006) and later through the creation of 'The Stepping Model' by Norton et al. (2020) and their subsequent discussions on informality, specifically by Norton et al. (2023).

Professionalism arises from the Peer Support Worker's obligation to abide by the terms and conditions of their employment in their respective organisations – statutory services or non-governmental associations (NGOs). However, friendship is evident through several means including the place in which peer support activities occur and indeed the sharing of one's lived experiences and the subsequent trust that is built from these factors. In essence, the mechanism required to create informality has the side effect of creating what seems to be something like that of a friendship. However, this is not a typical friendship as due to the professional background of the service that employs Peer Support Workers as well as the discipline that is created by formalised peers themselves, the relationship created is friend-like. Friend-like relationships carry aspects of a genuine friendship, but the caveat is that there are clear boundaries attached. The idea of ethical informality is raised because of the lack of clarity as to how informality can be present in the same space as such boundaries outlined here.

When one explores the concept of friendship in the workplace context, the narrative enters a complex area. In a seminal study of friendship by Spencer and Pahl (2006), they present a table examining the differences and similarities between that of friend and that of family. In a later study conducted by Bates (2021), two further columns were added representing that of the befriender and staff to explore the differences between same (Table 8.1).

It is important to understand the distinction between these concepts for several reasons. Firstly, the staff's potential use of an informal friendship could cause ambiguity between actual informal friendship, family and other community relationships. For instance, a person with an enduring mental health challenge calls the staff who work in their hostel, their friend. When this occurs, and disagreements follow, staff could resort to their default position and offer service solutions rather than supporting the person to engage with their community. Perhaps most worrying is the possibility of the service user thinking that because of this improper use of friend-like relationships by staff such formally constrained relationships are appropriate for all other human connections. This can have the devastating impact of weakening the person's ability to interact with actual friends on an informal basis. Of further importance to note when speaking of ethical informality is what happens at a specific point in the peer support relationship. For instance, for many professional staff, their relationship with the service user commences with a referral, however, for some peers, their connection with the service user begins much earlier, perhaps when both the peer and service user were fellow inpatients on a psychiatric ward. Such prior relationships are not uncommon but are more frequent for Peer Support Workers. However, no literature has yet discussed how to navigate a relationship with such a non-formal history.

Table 8.1 Befriending Is More Like a Staff Relationship than a Friendship

	Family	Friend	Befriender	Staff
Choice	A given relationship	A chosen relationship	An arranged relationship	An assigned relationship
Responsibility	Mutual obligation, more on elders	Cannot expect obligation	Boundaries might be set	Clear rules for conducting relationship
Importance	Taken for granted	Linked to quality of relatioship	Project oversees Commitment	Duty on staff to deliver support
Continuity	Expected to survive ups and downs	May not last	Continues while project approves	Expected to end when task achieved
Affection	Expected to love each other	Expected to like each other	Duty on befriender to try	Staff must respect the client

8.3 Working in an Environment Where One Was Formally a Patient

Peer Support Workers are lived experience professionals who have a past lived experience of mental health challenges and subsequent recovery (Viking et al., 2022; Gillard et al., 2024). Their inclusion within traditional mental health structures is a powerful catalyst towards the broader aim of services to become recovery-orientated (Naughton et al., 2015). In this way, the presence and work of the peer is extremely meaningful (Wall et al., 2022). However, when initially planning for the introduction of Peer Support Workers in traditional systems, careful consideration of such planning is necessary to provide an emotional and physical sense of safety for the peer and the individuals they are employed to support (Repper et al., 2019). This is also extremely important as peers, if their implementation is not planned correctly could end up on a team that treated them in the past or in an environment by which they were an inpatient/outpatient during their own recovery journey. This situation can cause an ethical challenge as the peer in this instance immediately transforms from a person the staff in such settings supported a colleague. In Case Study 8, Nina describes how she worked as a peer in the same ward as she was an inpatient.

Case Study 8   Peer Support in an Emergency Inpatient Ward in Iceland

Nina Eck

Implementation of peer support in the Icelandic National Hospital started in recovery wards. I remember when the nurse manager of the acute inpatient ward requested that I work there as a peer. When I had applied for the job months earlier, I had hoped to be able to travel back to my own inpatient stay to tell myself that recovery was possible for me. This was my opportunity to give that image of hope to those currently struggling.

Emergency inpatient wards are places where people with a lot of emotional pain go to seek respite from their environment and alleviation of their suffering. For people experiencing their first inpatient stay, it is also a place where they have to come to terms with the fact that they now belong to a marginalised group. For myself, this change to my self-image was one of the most defining moments of my life. Looking back, this is something I dedicated my working life to helping people through.

My first shift on that ward was a mixture of excitement and fear. I was excited to give back to the invaluable nurse that had shown me respect and kindness in my inpatient stay four years earlier, excited to try something new and use my experience to relate to those currently struggling. My anxiety and fear was related to my position as a former patient in the ward. Hanging out in the nurses station felt alien and seeing patient notes felt like an invasion of a friend's privacy. I was so scared that the staff would see me as a patient but at the same time scared that the residents would see me as a normal member of staff.

The ward is laid out in a big, L' shape, the nurses station being in the bend between two hallways of rooms. Common areas consisted of an open dining area, a TV nook with a puzzle area and a little room with a computer and some colouring books. In the beginning, I would sit in the TV area or dining area depending on where there were more people. For clarification, I talk about, patients' as people and staff members as such. As someone staying in inpatient, there is already so much going on that removes your humanity and I want to do my part in giving it back to them. In the ward, I would sometimes try to insert myself into conversations but most often I would just be visible and wait for people to come up to me and ask me what I'm doing.

Emergency inpatient stays are commonly seen as an emergency medical intervention. Although it is often a deeply personal and sometimes traumatic experience for people. They are put into an environment where they lose their privacy, the ability to decide how they spend their day, and sometimes their right to self-determination. They share an unlockable room with a stranger that has a windowed door so staff can peek in at all times. Staff's access to residents is uninhibited, but for them to access staff they need to knock on the door of the nurses station and make a request. Smokers cannot decide when they smoke themselves, which often adds to their anxiety. Phone chargers are kept in the nurses station because they can be used for self-harm purposes. The environment is 'safe' and reminds people constantly that they're not allowed to take their own lives. On top of all this, the ward often houses over 20 people in distress, which can also have an impact on them.

Forming that initial connection to people was difficult at the beginning. They were not used to having conversations about anything other than their problems or symptoms, in addition to the role of peer being unheard of. Often I had to explain that I could not assist them in obtaining medication, I could not get utensils from the locked kitchen and that I could not make decisions about whether or not they could go out to smoke. I realised pretty quickly that I had to think about my appearance. People regularly asked me if I was working there, since I was the only one apart from the psychologists and social workers that wasn't wearing scrubs. I always wore a lanyard that identified me as a member of staff but was never running around or busy like my coworkers. While conversing with people for the first time I often felt like there was a barrier I had to break through so they would see me as different from other staff. The fastest and most effective way to do that is to overshare about my own experience, but other methods included wearing orange grip socks, eating meals with people (not in the staff dining hall), and asking the residents practical questions about staying in the ward. Questions like where to find said socks, what recreational activities were planned for the day, where to find a pen and so on.

At one point in time I had assistance in forming connections. Someone staying in the ward who was in a state labelled mania. They were talking a lot, pacing, listening to and showing others music and poetry. I formed a good connection with them during a short shift and then came back a couple of days later. In the meantime, they had told everyone staying in the ward about me and my role. When I walked into the ward those days later, the person pulled a small group of people together and introduced me to them. This experience made me realise I had been unfairly prejudiced against people in a state similar to theirs. I really felt like they had done the hardest part of my job for me while I wasn't even there.

My role as the first peer in that ward was to figure out how a peer fits into the daily routine of the ward, to help healthcare professionals recognise who might benefit from a conversation with a peer, what support the peer brings to residents, and where the peer fits on the spectrum between residents and staff. Some wards have slow starts in the morning but in this one, many people are already up and about by the time the morning shift shows up. The population can also give important information on the personality of the perfect peer. In this particular ward there is a wide age gap of people, from young women experiencing rejection to older people in mental distress. The people staying there often don't stay for long, so the ward would benefit from a peer coming regularly as to be able to meet as many as possible.

Today the ward employs their own peer. The staff are aware of the service she can offer and will recommend she introduce herself to some people they've identified as needing a peer. They will also talk about her to people so they might seek her out when she comes. The peer is an older woman with a background as a school teacher. This means that she can take on a warm motherly role to the younger individuals and can connect to the older residents in a unique way. She is part of the multidisciplinary team working there but has a unique role as a cultural broker, bridging the gap between professionals and those staying in the ward. Part of her job is also to instil hope in those finding themselves at a hopeless point in their life, but the core of the role revolves around building human connection. Our peers are trained in the art of connection and building equal relationships through Intentional Peer Support, which not only helps them connect to others, but first connecting to themselves.

Since starting her work there a year and a half ago, she has already identified the times and circumstances when her presence is most useful to the people and the ward. She takes active part in pointing out where the ward and its staff need to do better for their target group. The ward staff talks highly about her both to people coming in, and to other staff within the hospital. She is an advocate for the people she works with and has said that through her long employment history, this is the job she receives the most praise for.

Although Nina's experience was positive, she has noted issues in terms of her identity as a peer and as a member of staff and how to break down barriers to her work with inpatients on the ward. She also highlighted that she wanted to make the nurse who helped her over the course of her own mental health challenges proud. Although her experience was positive, the ethical issue of being placed in an environment where one was formerly an inpatient raised its head again. Through Nina's past experiences with this nurse, Nina may feel under pressure to deliver results to impress this nurse, thereby putting the interests of the patient secondary to that of this particular nurse. Additionally, Nina mentions the access to patient notes. This may raise an ethical concern if a relative or close friend comes into the ward as an inpatient. In such a scenario, she may have undue access to clinical information that inherently breaches a person's privacy. However, it is important to note that in Nina's scenario above, the result of her working there was positive as this ward continues to employ peers into their system. Indeed, this ethical concern is one of a multitude of reasons why supervision of the role is vitally important (Daniels et al., 2015; Watson et al., 2024). However, as we will now discover, supervision within peer support work also raises issues which need further exploration. Section 8.4, which explores these issues is now presented.

8.4 The Supervision of Peers

There is an increasing number of calls for action in relation to Peer Support Workers being supervised by their own discipline (Mahon and Sharek, 2024; Norton et al., 2023a). However, these calls come relatively unanswered due to the infancy of the peer support profession. Although there are signs of this becoming reality in Ireland with the establishment of the Senior Peer Support Worker role, the suspicions of other professionals, particularly psychiatry into the appropriate use of peer support in mental health is another reason why such calls have remained relatively unanswered till this point (Mahon and Norton, 2024). As a result, it is now timely that the discussions had in this book and elsewhere are happening.

Within health and social care, supervision forms a central component of the work (O'Donnell, 2015; Rothwell et al., 2021) There are several benefits to both the individual and organisation for regular supervision to occur. Firstly, supervision allows for an individual's performance to be reviewed and if necessary adjusted and modified for the betterment of the organisation (Care Council for Wales, 2012). On an individual basis, it allows the worker the time and space to reflect on previous practices so that if such an event happens again, the individual is more equipped to deal with it. Organisationally, supervision is linked to improvements in practice which results in better outcomes and less strain inflicted upon the health services (Health Service Executive, 2019). Despite these benefits, there remains a lack of commitment towards implementing robust processes and structures for supervision within health care.

Within Irish services, Peer Support Workers have been in place since 2017. However, as the role progressed, an identified need for specific supervision within the discipline has grown due to issues of role clarity and the therapeutic use of lived experiences to aid recovery whilst in the role (Norton, 2022).[2] This has raised flags within the peer profession as for some, there is a belief that the authenticity of peer support work is being infringed upon and weakened as a direct result of being supervised by a different discipline which ultimately comes from a different epistemological position to that of the peer (Norton, 2023; Norton et al., 2023a). This has been discussed in a previous chapter and work remains on rectifying this dilemma through the introduction of Senior Peer Support Workers or supervisory equivalents within mental health services nationally and internationally. Despite this promising development, it is too early to say whether the issues portrayed in this book will be rectified by the introduction of such positions into mental health service provision and discourse.

8.4.1   Current Supervision in Peer Support Work – From a Peer's Perspective

In Irish mental health services – where I practised as a Peer Support Worker between 2017 and 2020 – such employees are supervised as well as line managed by the discipline of social work (Griffin, 2022). For me, this has presented both challenges and solutions to issues that have arisen over the years. The model of supervision that was created by social work is one aspect that peers have been extremely lucky to inherit as it focuses on the person's practice, their own development and their self-care. This model of supervision is the Morrison (2005) 4×4×4 model (Figure 8.2). It is a useful approach to supervision as it takes

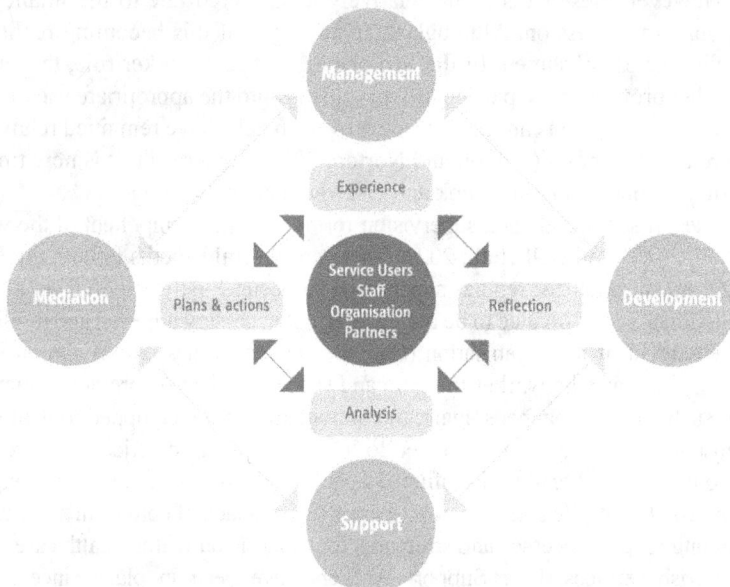

Figure 8.2 Morrison's 4×4×4 Supervision Model.

into account a number of different processes whilst also being strengths-based (Maglailic, 2020).

Within supervision, the peer is expected and encouraged to form the agenda as well as note-taking during the session. The notes are taken on a template like that presented in Appendix and are based on Morrison's 4×4×4 model to structure the supervision session. For me, supervision always commences with a wellness check. This is useful in identifying if the peer is in a space where they can openly reflect, without judgement on their experiences (Mahon and Norton, 2024). After this, the supervisor goes through the various aspects of the form as a guide for various discussions. Once supervision concludes, it is my responsibility as the supervisee to type up the notes, follow up on agreed actions and send the signed minutes to the supervisor for their approval and signature. This document is then placed and stored within the employee file and only brought out again if there is a disagreement or if a matter arising needs checking as it pertains to the practice of the peer.

8.5 The Training of the Peer Support Worker

As Peer Support Workers are identified as a unique discipline within mental health discourse, they require specific training to undertake certain roles and functions effectively so that they can provide support effectively (Norton et al., 2023b). Indeed, the training of peers is considered an essential component in supporting individuals in their preparations to become formalised Peer Support Workers (Repper et al., 2013; Griffin et al., 2024). Consequently, certified training in this area is now a necessary criterion for organisations like the Health Service Executive to request when recruiting service users for the role (Repper et al., 2013). When it comes to the content of such training, there is no rule book. However, peers are expected to be trained in a culturally responsive and trauma-informed manner (Pachowicz and Goffe, 2024). A recent paper by Sanchez-Moscona and Eiroa-Orosa (2021) identified a number of modules that should be compulsory for any certified training being supplied to future peers (Table 8.2).

Along with the modules identified by Sanchez-Moscona and Eiroa-Orosa (2021) in Table 8.2, Machin (2019) also identified that any certified training of the peer should aim to achieve the following learning outcomes:

1. To explore the background of peer support inclusive of social justice, service user activism and the recovery movement,
2. To explore the core values of peer support work,
3. To identify and critically examine the setting in which peer support work occurs inclusive of the needs of the organisation as well as the wider community,
4. To identify and enhance self-care practices, boundary setting and safe disclosure and,
5. To learn and enhance peer support work's core skills inclusive of active listening, expression of lived experience and managing challenging situations.

(Machin, 2019)

Table 8.2 Mandatory Modules in Peer Support Worker Training

Module	Description
Pedagogy Applied to Recovery	Approaches to mental health recovery, key concepts and factors involved.
Participatory Methodologies	Using the previous sessions and expanding on the same. Learning about recovery as a unique process, its history, what promotes recovery, CHIME framework.
Group Dynamics	Management of group dynamics introduced, Maslow's Hierarchy of Needs, emotional intelligence, facilitation skills.
Role Playing	Introduction to tools used to facilitate learning of theoretical and applied content, analysing self and others behaviour, basics of peer support working.
Accompaniment and Mutual Aid Groups	Forms of peer support, recovery values/principles, accompanying and communication skills, ethical codes.
Rights	Tools to respect service user's rights, wills and preferences, advanced directives, legalities – Rights of the Person with Disabilities.
Language and Communication	Language skills to establish respectful and mutual relationships with service users, mastering verbal and non-verbal communication cues.
Risks and Limits	Ethical principles, sensitive issues and risks – self-harm, suicidal ideation and intent detected.
Comparisons of Training Models	Comparing training models of other countries/jurisdictions

Source: Extracted from Sanchez-Moscona and Eiroa-Orosa (2021).

Within an Irish context, there are currently two sites where the training of Peer Support Workers and Family Peer Support Workers[3] occur: Dublin City University (DCU)[4] and Atlantic Technological University (ATU), Castlebar Campus.[5] The course in DCU, like in ATU runs over the course of one year and results in a level 8 special purpose award in peer support working. The idea behind the duration of the courses is that the student themselves comes to the training with lived experiences of mental health challenges and recovery. This experiential expertise is weighed as equivalent to three years of undergraduate study. The purpose of the one-year programme therefore is to support the peer in harnessing their inner expertise to support others in mental distress. Unlike ATU, DCU has a placement component lasting the entire year which allows students to embrace what they have learned and put it into practice. Currently, in the Irish health services, work is required to build capacity for such placement. Such work includes the development of Senior Peer Support Workers and addressing the governance-related risk concerns that are well established in the system. As a result, students often attain a placement with a non-governmental organisation (NGO) to meet these placement hours. This inherently causes significant barriers when it comes to hiring peers as they have little to no experience of working on a multi-disciplinary team and dependent on the original placement, may not have access before service users in acute distress.

In ATU, students can choose to specialise in a sub-discipline including addiction, neurodiversity or peer support for dementia and declining cognitive functioning. This is an important element of peer training as it helps steer the path for certain specialisms to be created in the future.[6] This has already begun with the creation of the Family Peer Support Worker[7] and by recent enquiries from the forensic mental health services in regards to acquiring Peer Support Workers in an Irish context. As a result, what is certain is that the discipline of peer support is quickly growing both in Ireland and internationally and as such this will require amendments to training as the evidence base to peer support itself evolves.

8.6 Concluding Remarks

To conclude, this chapter examined the ethical implications of the practice of peer support work. We first examined the dual role created as a direct result of the formation of informality. The '*professional/friend*' role is imperative for peer support work to be therapeutic but does raise ethical questions regarding how to be both a '*professional*' and '*friend*' at the same time. We then examined the ethical implications of being an employee of a service that the peer would have used when they were in mental distress followed by the ethical consideration regarding being supervised by a professional with a different epistemological position to that of the peer. Lastly, we explored the training of the peer and how it focuses on the therapeutic use of lived expertise and how in Ireland at present, there are inconsistencies in how Peer Support Workers are trained, leading to issues being formed in recruitment and practice. In the next chapter, we yet again move on from this discussion to explore whether peers being involved in traditional multi-disciplinary teams is the correct path for implementation or not. If this is not the case, the chapter will also explore what other avenues are available.

Notes

1 Chapter 7.
2 See Chapter 6 for more details.
3 To be explored in Chapter 11.
4 www.dcu.ie/courses/undergraduate/school-nursing-psychotherapy-and-community-health/certificate-peer-support
5 www.atu.ie/courses/certificate-peer-support-practice
6 See Chapter 12 for more details.
7 See Chapter 11 for more details.

References

Barlow, C.A., Schiff, J.W., Chugh, U., Rawlinson, D., Hides, E. & Leith, J. (2010) An evaluation of a suicide bereavement peer support program. *Death Studies* 34(10), 915–930. https://doi.org/10.1080/07481181003761435

Bates, P. (2021) *Searching for Friendship in Befriending Schemes* (Internet). Available at: https://peterbates.org.uk/wp-content/uploads/2021/05/Searching-for-friendship-in-Befriending-Schemes.pdf (Accessed 14 January 2025).

Boardman, G., Kerr, D. & McCann, T. (2015) Peer experience of delivering a problem-solving programme to enhance antipsychotic medication adherence for individuals with schizophrenia. *Journal of Psychiatric and Mental Health Nursing* 22(6), 423–430. https://doi.org/10.1111/jpm.12195

Care Council for Wales (2012) *Supervising and Appraising Well: A Guide to Effective Supervision and Appraisal for those Working in Social Care* (Internet). Available at: https://socialcare.wales/cms-assets/documents/Supervising-and-appraising-well-social-care.pdf (Accessed 16 January 2025).

Daniels, A.S., Tunner, T.P., Powell, I., Fricks, L. & Ashenden, P. (2015) *Pillars of Peer Support Services Summit Six: Peer Specialist Supervision* (Internet). Available at: https://copelandcenter.com/sites/default/files/2024-02/POPS2014.pdf (Accessed 19 January 2025).

Davidson, L., Chinman, M., Sells, D. & Rowe, M. (2006) Peer support among adults with serious mental illness: A report from the field. *Schizophrenia Bulletin* 32(3), 443–450. https://doi.org/10.1093/schbul/sbj043

Faulkner, A. & Basset, T. (2010) *A Helping Hand: Consultations with Service Users about Peer Support* (Internet). Available at: www.together-uk.org/wp-content/uploads/2023/08/A-helping-hand-consultation-with-service-users-about-peer-support.pdf (Accessed 17 January 2025).

Gillard, S., Foster, R., White, S., Bhattacharya, R., Binfield, P., Eborall, R., Gibson, S.L., Harnett, D., Simpson, A., Lucock, M., Marks, J., Repper, J., Rinaldi, M., Salla, A. & Worner, J. (2024) Implementing peer support into practice in mental health services: A qualitative comparative case study. *BMC Health Services Research* 24, 1050. https://doi.org/10.1186/s12913-024-11447-5

Griffin, M. (2022) *Peer Support Working in Mental Health: A System in Need of Change?* (Internet). Available at: https://madinireland.com/2022/08/peer-support-working-in-mental-health-a-system-in-need-of-change/ (Accessed 19 January 2025).

Griffin, M., Duff, P. & MacGabhann, L. (2024) The training and education of peer support workers. In *Peer Support Work: Practice, Training and Implementation* (Mahon, D. ed.). Emerald Publishing Limited, Leeds, pp. 115–127.

Health Service Executive (2019) *Clinical Supervision for Nurses Working in Mental Health Services: A Guide for Nurse Managers, Supervisors and Supervisees* (Internet). Available at: www.lenus.ie/bitstream/handle/10147/626949/clinical%20supervision%20for%20nurses%20working%20in%20mental%20health%20services%20a%20guide%20%20final.pdf?sequence=1 (Accessed 16 January 2025).

Machin, K. (2019) Peer support training. In *Peer Support in Mental Health* (Watson, E. & Meddings, S. eds.). Red Globe Press, London, pp. 99–113.

Maglailic, R.A. (2020) *PSDP – Resources and Tools: The Role and Function of Supervision* (Internet). Available at: https://practice-supervisors.rip.org.uk/wp-content/uploads/2020/11/KB_The_role_and_functions_of_supervision_NEW.pdf (Accessed 16 January 2025).

Mahon, D. & Norton, M.J. (2024) The supervision of peers. In *Peer Support Work: Practice, Training and Implementation* (Mahon, D. ed.). Emerald Publishing Limited, Leeds, pp. 105–114.

Mahon, D. & Sharek, D. (2024) An exploration of the implementation of peer work across multiple fields in Ireland. *Mental Health and Social Inclusion* 28(5), 485–504. https://doi. org/10.1108/MHSI-12-2022-0082

Morison T. (2005) *Staff Supervision in Social Care*. Pavilion Publishing, Brighton.

Naughton, L., Collins, P. & Ryan, M. (2015) *Peer Support Workers: A Guidance Paper* (Internet). Available at: www.hse.ie/eng/services/list/4/mental-health-services/men talhealthengagement/peer-support-workers-a-guidance-paper.pdf   (Accessed   19 January 2025).

Norton, M.J. (2022) More than just a health care assistant: Peer support working within rehabilitation and recovery mental health services. *Irish Journal of Psychological Medicine*. https://doi.org/10.1017/ipm.2022.32

Norton, M.J. (2023) Peer support working: A question of ontology and epistemology? *International Journal of Mental Health Systems* 17, 1. https://doi.org/10.1186/s13 033-023-00570-1

Norton, M.J., Archard, P. & Swords, C. (2023) The ethics of informality and dual rela-tionships in peer support. *Psychiatric Services* 74(2), 2. https://doi.org/10.1176/appi. ps.20230291

Norton, M.J., Bergin, M. & Denieffe, S. (2020) *Service User Views of Peer Support in Mental Health: A Systematic Review and Meta-Synthesis*. Unpublished Manuscript.

Norton, M.J., Clabby, P., Coyle, B., Cruickshank, J., Davidson, G., Greer, K., Kilcommins, M., McCartan, C., McGuire, E., McGilloway, S., Mulholland, C., Oconnell-Gannon, M., Pepper, D., Shannon, C., Swords, C., Walsh, J. & Webb, P. (2023) *Peer Support Work: An International Scoping Review – Summary Report* (Internet). Available at: https://puread min.qub.ac.uk/ws/portalfiles/portal/543700214/Peer_Support_Work_Scoping_Rev iew_Main_report.pdf (Accessed 19 January 2025).

Norton, M.J., Griffin, M., Collins, M., Clark, M. & Browne, E. (2023a) Using autoeth-nography to reflect on peer support supervision in an Irish context. *Journal of Practice Teaching and Learning* 20(1–2). https://doi.org/10.1921/jpts.v21i2.2079

O'Donnell, J. (2015) *Supervision among Social Care Workers: Prevalence and Effect*. Masters Dissertation, Athlone Institute of Technology, Athlone, Ireland.

Pachowicz, M. & Goffe, A. (2024) *Family Peer Support Work: A Review of Irish and International Literature* (Internet). Available at: www.tasc.ie/assets/files/pdf/family_peer _support_work_november_2024.pdf (Accessed 19 January 2025).

Repper, J., Aldridge, B., Gilfoyle, S., Gillard, S., Perkins, R. & Rennison, J. (2013) *Peer Support Workers: A Practical Guide to Implementation* (Internet). Available at: https:// static1.squarespace.com/static/65e873c27971d37984653be0/t/668ce1d012bd721c16847 151/1720508881816/7-Peer-Support-Workers a-practical-guide-to-implementation.pdf (Accessed 19 January 2025).

Repper, J., Walker, L., Skinner, S. & Ball, M. (2019) *Preparing Organisations for Peer Support: Creating a Culture and Context in Which Peer Support Workers Thrive* (Internet). Available at: https://static1.squarespace.com/static/65e873c27971d37984653be0/t/668c0 afdb379ec78d6f680fd/1720453887036/17ImROC-Preparing-Organisations-PSW-Brief ing-Paper-1.pdf (Accessed 19 January 2025).

Rothwell, C., Kehoe, A., Farook, S.F. & Illing, J. (2021) Enablers and barriers to effective clinical supervision in the workplace: A rapid evidence review. *BMJ Open* 11(9), e052929. https://doi.org/10.1136/bmjopen-2021-052929

Sanchez-Moscona, C. & Eiroa-Orosa, F.J. (2021) Training mental health peer support training facilitators: A qualitative, participatory evaluation. *International Journal of Mental Health Nursing* 30(1), 261–273. https://doi.org/10.1111/inm.12781

Shaw, L., Sumison, T., Moll, S., Holmes, J., Geronimo, J. & Sherman, D. (2009) Work transitions for peer support providers in traditional mental health programs: Unique challenges and opportunities. *Work: A Journal of Prevention, Assessment and Rehabilitation* 33(4), 449–458. https://doi.org/10.3233/WOR-2009-0893

Smedberg, M.B. (2015) *The Integration of Peer Support Specialists: A Qualitative Study.* Masters Thesis, St Catherine University and the University of St Thomas, Minnesota, United States of America.

Spencer, L. & Pahl, R. (2006) *Rethinking Friendship: Hidden Solidarities Today.* Princeton University Press, New Jersey.

Viking, T., Wenzer, J., Hylin, U. & Nilsson, L. (2022) Peer support workers' role and expertise and interprofessional learning in mental health care: A scoping review. *Journal of Interprofessional Care* 36(6), 828–838. https://doi.org/10.1080/13561820.2021.2014796

Walker, G. & Bryant, W. (2013) Peer support in adult mental health services: A metasynthesis of qualitative findings. *Psychiatric Rehabilitation Journal* 36(1), 28–34. https://doi.org/10.1037/h0094744

Wall, A., Lovheden, T., Landgren, K. & Stjernsward, S. (2022) Experiences and challenges in the role as peer support worker in a Swedish mental health context – An interview study. *Issues in Mental Health Nursing* 43(4), 344–355. https://doi.org/10.1080/01612840.2021.1978596

Watson, E., Bowyer, D., Cooper, S., Dodd, Z., Manning, E., Morgan, G., Owen, D., Repper, J., Repper, P. & Szmit, D. (2024) *Supervision of Peer Workers* (Internet). Available at: https://static1.squarespace.com/static/65e873c27971d37984653be0/t/66b344308706157585716563/1723024432598/ImROC+Briefing+Paper+25+%283%29.pdf (Accessed 19 January 2025).

Appendix: Sample Peer Supervision Record Template

Pro Forma – Supervision Record for Staff File

Record of Supervision Meeting Held on Date:			
Supervisee Name:			
Supervisor Name:			
Supervision Area	**Actions Agreed**	**By Whom**	**When**
Management and Case Discussion			
Professional Development			
Support			
Engagement			
AOB			
Record of Any Disagreement			

Signature _____

Supervisor _____ Date: _____

Signature

Chapter 9

Peer Support Work in Traditional Mental Health Discourse

9.1 Introduction

In the previous chapter of this text, ethical issues as it pertains to peer support work were identified and critically discussed. These ethical challenges, particularly as they relate to that of the dual role, creation of informality and working in a system where one was formally a patient all point towards an argument to be made as to whether Peer Support Workers should be placed within traditional mental health service provision or be situated external to this. In this chapter, I aim to examine this argument in detail drawing from the latest evidence in the field. This will take place in Section 9.2. After which, Section 9.3 will conclude the chapter with my personal perspective on this question.

9.2 The Placement of the Peer Support Worker in Traditional Mental Health Services

Mental health services are increasingly implementing Peer Support Workers into traditional service discourse (Trachtenberg et al., n.d.; Fortuna et al., 2022). With this comes both opportunities and challenges that not only impact the multi-disciplinary team that takes on the peer but also the Peer Support Worker themselves (Poremski et al., 2022; Haun et al., 2024). In recent articles by both Almeida et al., (2020) and Lerbaek et al. (2024), they identified that the Peer Support Worker workforce in particular has been the fastest-growing professional discipline in the history of mental health service provision. Part of the rationale for such endorsement and growth within the traditional service space is the Peer Support Workers' ability to effectively promote a recovery-orientated culture within a traditional health organisation (Lerbaek et al., 2024). Despite evidence to suggest that the implementation of Peer Support Worker was indeed successful (Gillard et al., 2014), the integration of these posts within traditional discourse has not come without its challenges, which include the impact the role has on the peer itself. Such challenges require serious consideration so that they do not impede the future development of the role (Gillard and Holley, 2014; Kilpatrick et al., 2017; Poremski et al., 2022; Grim et al., 2023). Despite this warning for immediate attention, to date, there has been

DOI: 10.4324/9781032717050-12

a paucity of debate surrounding the effects working in this environment has on the Peer Support Workers themselves (Klingemann et al., 2024). What little data is out there is often contradictory. For example, Gillard et al., (2022) found that peers were no more likely to encounter negative impacts of working in the health system than any other type of healthcare professional. This contradicts with other authors in the field who noted unique challenges to the peer such as emotional burden, moral distress leading to poor treatment of the Peer Support Worker by the system, getting caught up on systemic power imbalances and the eventual co-optation of the peer (Watson and Repper n.d.; Miyamoto and Sono, 2012; Griffin, 2022; Klingemann et al., 2024; Cooper et al., 2025).

But what parameters set successful implementation of the role that does not risk a peer's emotional and moral integrity? According to Ehrlich et al. (2020) success-ful integration of Peer Support Workers onto the multi-disciplinary teams is totally dependent on the ability of traditional staff to focus on the strengths the peer brings to the team beyond that of lived experience itself. Robertson et al. (2024) add to this by suggesting that the likelihood of burnout within peer support is also dependent on the level of support given by the line manager/supervisor as well as that of the multi-disciplinary team. However, Gillard (2019) suggests that issues of implemen-tation and acceptance into the role may be a side argument of a much bigger ques-tion policy makers as well as peers need to ask themselves. According to Gillard (2019), the real question to ask is whether peer support work is philosophically, therapeutically and theoretically the same when it is taken from the informal, mutual environment of informal peer support and moved to an environment that represents the mental health services, which is noted by Gillard as contrived and constrained.

As already noted in this text, the idea of peer support is neither new nor lim-ited to mental health service provision (Davidson et al., 2018). Regardless of the situation of the concept, peer support work is noted to be based upon the premise that those who have endured and overcome a challenge can and do offer support, encouragement and hope to those facing similar challenges (Schon, 2010). Within mental health service provision, peer support work should not be viewed as an alternative approach, but instead, it should be observed as a necessary, comple-mentary aspect to that of usual care (Firsthand, n.d.; Kuhn et al., 2015). When it comes to the professionalisation of the peer role in mental health discourse, the system that professionalises them has received much scrutiny as this diminishes the powerful impact the informal, spontaneous and naturally occurring phenomena have on those in an earlier phase of recovery (Repper et al., 2013). Penny (2018) adds to this discussion by suggesting Peer Support Workers by means of profes-sionalisation cannot perform true 'peer support' due to the hierarchical boundaries that are invisibly there during their work with service users. Instead, Penny argues that these peers usually just disclose their lived experiences, which result a role-modelling function for the people they are employed to serve (Penny, 2018). This idea of the inability to create pure mutuality is seconded by Davidson et al. (2006) who also suggests that the same rule applies to that of reciprocity. As a result, Chinman et al. (2014) suggest that this relationship actually turns asymmetrical leading to something different than peer support coming into play. As such, Penny (2018) states that this results in the use of the term 'peer' as a euphemism for service users is philosophically problematic. However, Penny (2018) does not offer a resolution for this asymmetrical relationship and philosophical discourse.

Another area of growing concern is that the Peer Support Worker could get exploited by the system they work within to provide the same status quo service but at a much lower cost (Davidson, 2014). An example of this is noted by Norton, (2022, 2024) when he suggests that peers may appear to do the same role or utilise the same instruments as other professionals, but in fact, these tasks and tools are transformed into something new due to the application of experiential knowledge to the task, tool and role. However, this still raises concern amongst academics who write in this field and the knowledge as to the transformation discussed above is only now slowly beginning to emerge.

Additionally, services take on the Peer Support Worker role often tokenistically to show that they are becoming recovery-orientated (Davidson, 2014). However, this assumption is impossible in some respects as ideologically, Peer Support Workers work from a different compass to that of other service providers on the multi-disciplinary team (Chapman et al., 2018). The Peer Support Worker works on the assumption of recovery as a re-enchantment with life, an opportunity to reflect, grow and live well with illness (Anthony, 1993; Watts 2012; Norton and Cullen, 2024a). This differs from the non-peer mental health professional who operates under a biopsychosocial approach which essentially advocates for the elimination of signs and symptoms of mental illness and the gradual rehabilitation of service users back to a previous level of functioning (Slade and Longden, 2015). In this way, the work of the peer, on an ideological level, clashes with that of other service providers as the peer sees a life for the service user even with the limitations that are caused by illness. In this way, peers recognise that 'illness' is formed as a result of trauma and as such never truly leaves an individual (Norton and Cullen, 2024b). Instead, the person affected morphs and grows around the limitations that trauma holds on the person. Other providers may recognise trauma, but still inherently rely on the idea that recovery is the complete elimination of signs and symptoms of 'illness' and a return to functioning. The peer notes that a return to functioning is not possible, rather this functioning is built further in time as the person learns to live with their condition and live a hopeful, satisfying and contributing life despite the presence of 'illness'. As such, the two cannot and should not co-exist within the one service.

In summary, the implementation and integration challenges noted (the lack of pure mutuality and reciprocity, the potential of exploitation of the Peer Support Worker, the ideological conflicts between the recovery movement and more traditional biopsychosocial cultures as well as the professionalisation of the peer) within mental health service provision are all rationales as to why the professional, formalised Peer Support Worker placement within a traditional mental health service may not be the correct move for policy makers when considering implementing the role (Simpson et al., 2017; Shalaby and Agyapong, 2020). However, it is noted that this area of scholarship is currently poorly examined and as such, future studies should explore the issues raised here more thoroughly to create a final decision as to whether the placement of Peer Support Workers in traditional mental health services is indeed the right decision for all involved.

9.3 Concluding Remarks

This chapter examined the debate as to whether Peer Support Workers should work within a mental health service or external to it. Not surprisingly, the evidence in this area of peer support scholarship is sparse to say the least. A rationale for this is that to date, academic inquiry has only focussed on testing its impact and feasibility within mental health discourse with little literature exploring issues of implementation, integration and the philosophical placement of the peer. It is interesting to find that the literature base is starting to suggest that the Peer Support Worker should not be in traditional systems due to issues of hierarchy, moral injury and professionalism. My own thoughts on this, as a former Peer Support Worker and individual who has managed the implementation of peers in Ireland, is that I see these issues arising daily in my work. I see peers who are for one reason or another struggling with the system in place. Equally, I also see peers who are doing phenomenal work in the area. The key difference between peers who are struggling and peers who are striving is organisational commitment. The peers who are satisfied in their role are the individuals who come from regional healthcare organisations that accept the recovery movement and have the backing of senior management who actually care about their employees and the lives of the end user. The opposite can be said for the areas in which peers are struggling. As such, I believe that Peer Support Workers have the ability to positively impact people's lives, both personally and organisationally. As such, I believe that peers can and should be placed within traditional structures, despite such ideological challenges noted, but only if the organisation is truly ready and committed to embracing peer work and its uniqueness within mental health service provision. One way to ensure organisational readiness is through the correct implementation of policy relating to the peer. This exact issue is the focus of the next chapter of this text.

References

Almeida, M., Day, A., Smith, B., Bianco, C. & Fortuna, K. (2020) Actionable items to address challenges incorporating peer support specialists within an integrated mental health and substance use disorder system: Co-designed qualitative study. *Journal of Participatory Medicine* 12(4), e17053. https://doi.org/10.2196/17053

Anthony, W.A. (1993) Recovery from mental illness: The guiding vision of the mental health service system in the 1990s. *Psychosocial Rehabilitation Journal* 16(4), 11–23. https://doi.org/10.1037/h0095655

Chapman, S.A., Blash, L.K., Mayer, K. & Spetz, J. (2018) Emerging roles for peer providers in mental health and substance use disorders. *American Journal of Preventive Medicine* 54(6), S267–S274. https://doi.org/10.1016/j.amepre.2018.02.019

Chinman, M., George, P., Dougherty, R.H., Daniels, A.S., Ghose, S.S., Swift, A. & Delphin-Rittmon, M.E. (2014) Peer support services for individuals with serious mental illnesses: Assessing the evidence. *Psychiatric Services* 65(4), 429–441. https://doi.org/10.1176/appi.ps.201300244

Cooper, R.E., Lyons, N., Nicholls, V., Foye, U., Shah, P., Mitchell, L., Machin, K., Chipp, B., Grundy, A., Pemovska, T., Ahmed, N., Appleton, R., Repper, J., Lloyd-Evans, B., Simpson, A. & Johnson, S. (2025) *Understanding the Roles and Experiences of Mental Health Peer Support Workers in England: A Qualitative Study* (Internet). Available at: www.medrxiv.org/content/10.1101/2025.01.16.25320547v1.article-info (Accessed 27 January 2025).

Davidson, L. (2014) *Peer Support in Mental Health: Exploitive, Transformative, or Both?* (Internet). Available at: www.madinamerica.com/2014/09/peer-support-mental-health-exploitive-transformative/#:~:text=The%20answer%20to%20which%20I,struggling%20with%20mental%20health%20issues (Accessed 27 January 2025).

Davidson, L., Bellamy, C., Chinman, M., Farkas, M., Ostrow, L., Cook, J.A., Jonikas, J.A., Rosenthal, H., Bergeson, S., Daniels, A.S. & Salzer, M. (2018) Revisiting the rationale and evidence for peer support. *Psychiatric Times* 35(6), 11–12.

Davidson, L., Chinman, M., Sells, D. & Rowe, M. (2006) Peer support among adults with serious mental illness: A report from the field. *Schizophrenia Bulletin* 32(3), 443–450. https://doi.org/10.1093/schbul/sbj043

Ehrlich, C., Slattery, M., Vilic, G., Chester, P. & Crompton, D. (2020) What happens when peer support workers are introduced as members of community-based clinical mental health service delivery teams: A qualitative study. *Journal of Interprofessional Care* 34(1), 107–115. https://doi.org/10.1080/13561820.2019.1612334

Firsthand (n.d.) *The Strength of Showing Up: How Peer Support Breaks the Mold of Traditional Care* (Internet). Available at: www.firsthandcares.com/blog/the-strength-of-showing-up#:~:text=The%20Transformative%20Power%20of%20Peer%20Support&text=Peers%20aren't%20perfect%2C%20but,are%20having%20a%20hard%20time (Accessed 27 January 2025).

Fortuna, K.L., Solomon, P. & Rivera, J. (2022) An update of peer support/peer provided services underlying processes, benefits, and critical ingredients. *Psychiatric Quarterly* 93, 571–586. https://doi.org/10.1007/s11126-022-09971-w

Gillard, S. (2019) Peer support in mental health services: Where is the research taking us, and do we want to go there? *Journal of Mental Health* 28(4), 341–344. https://doi.org/10.1080/09638237.2019.1608935

Gillard, S., Foster, R., White, S., Barlow, S., Bhattacharya, R., Binfield, P., Eborall, R., Faulkner, A., Gibson, S., Goldsmith, L.P., Simpson, A., Lucock, M., Marks, J., Morshead, R., Patel, S., Priebe, S., Repper, J., Rinaldi, M., Ussher, M. & Worner, J. (2022) The impact of working as a peer worker in mental health services: A longitudinal mixed methods study. *BMC Psychiatry* 22, 373. https://doi.org/10.1186/s12888-022-03999-9

Gillard, S., Foster, R., White, S., Bhattacharya, R., Binfield, P., Eborall, R., Gibson, S.L., Harnett, D., Simpson, A., Lucock, M., Marks, J., Repper, J., Rinaldi, M., Salla, A. & Worner, J. (2014) Implementing peer support into practice in mental health services: A qualitative comparative case study. *BMC Health Services Research* 24, 1050. https://doi.org/10.1186/s12913-024-11447-5

Gillard, S. & Holley, J. (2014) Peer workers in mental health services: Literature overview. *Advances in Psychiatric Treatment* 20, 286–292. https://doi.org/10.1192/apt.bp.113.011940

Griffin, M. (2022) *Peer Support Working in Mental Health: A System in Need of Change* (Internet). Available at: https://madinireland.com/2022/08/peer-support-working-in-men tal-health-a-system-in-need-of-change/ (Accessed 27 January 2025).

Grim, K., Bergmark, M., Argentzell, E. & Rosenberg, D. (2023) Managing peer support workers in Swedish mental health services – A leadership perspective on implementation and sustainability. *Journal of Psychosocial Rehabilitation and Mental Health* 10, 313–329. https://doi.org/10.1007/s40737-022-00311-6

Haun, M.H., Girit, S., Goldfarb, Y., Kalha, J., Korde, P., Kwebiiha, E., Moran, G., Mtei, R., Niwemuhwezi, J., Nixdorf, R., Nugent, L., Puschner, B., Ramesh, M., Ryan, G.K., Slade, M., Charles, A. & Krumm, S. (2024) Mental health workers' perspectives on the imple-mentation of a peer support intervention in five countries: Qualitative findings from the UPSIDES study. *BMJ Open* 14(5), e081963. https://doi.org/10.1136/bmjopen-2023-081963

Kilpatrick, E., Keeney, S. &McCauley, C.-O. (2017) Tokenistic or genuinely effective? Exploring the views of voluntary sector staff regarding the emerging peer support worker role in mental health. *Journal of Psychiatric and Mental Health Nursing* 24(7), 503–512. https://doi.org/10.1111/jpm.12391

Klingemann, J., Sienkiewicz-Jarosz, H., Molenda, B. & Switaj, P. (2024) Peer support work-ers in mental health services: A qualitative exploration of emotional burden, moral dis-tress and strategies to reduce the risk of mental health crisis. *Community Mental Health Journal*. https://doi.org/10.1007/s10597-024-01370-8

Kuhn, W., Bellinger, J., Stevens-Manser, S. & Kaufman, L. (2015) Integration of peer spe-cialists working in mental health service settings. *Community Mental Health Journal* 51, 453–458. https://doi.org/10.1007/s10597-015-9841-0

Lerbaek, B., Johansen, K., Burholt, A.K., Gregersen, L.M., Terp, M.O., Slade, M., Castelein, S. & Jorgensen, R. (2024) Non-peer professionals understanding of recovery and atti-tudes towards peer support workers joining existing community mental health teams in the north Denmark region: A qualitative study. *International Journal of Mental Health Nursing* 33(6), 2043–2053. https://doi.org/10.1111/inm.13349

Miyamoto, Y. & Sono, T. (2012) Lessons from peer support among individuals with mental health difficulties: A review of the literature. *Clinical Practice and Epidemiology in Mental Health* 8, 22–29.

Norton, M.J. (2022) More than just a health care assistant: Peer support working within rehabilitation and recovery mental health services. *Irish Journal of Psychological Medicine* 41(3), 420–421. https://doi.org/10.1017/ipm.2022.32

Norton, M.J. (2024) Using learned tools for experiential gain: The application of experien-tial knowledge to traditional service processes. *Irish Journal of Psychological Medicine*. https://doi.org/10.1017/ipm.2024.4

Norton, M.J. & Cullen, O.J. (2024a) Recovery in mental health, addiction and dual diag-nosis. In *Different Diagnoses, Similar Experiences: Narratives of Mental Health, Addiction Recovery and Dual Diagnosis* (Norton, M.J. & Cullen, O.J. eds.). Emerald Publishing Limited, Leeds, pp. 35–41.

Norton, M.J. & Cullen, O.J. (2024b) Fusing experiences, reflexive thematic analysis. In *Different Diagnoses, Similar Experiences: Narratives of Mental Health, Addiction Recovery and Dual Diagnosis* (Norton, M.J. & Cullen, O.J. eds.). Emerald Publishing Limited, Leeds, pp. 177–206.

Penny, D. (2018) *Defining 'Peer Support': Implications for Policy, Practice, and Research* (Internet). Available at: https://mamh-web.files.svdcdn.com/production/files/DPenney_ Defining_peer_support_2018_Final.pdf (Accessed 27 January 2025).

Poremski, D., Kuek, J.H.L., Yuan, Q., Li, Z., Yow, K.L., Eu, P.W. & Chua, H.C. (2022) The impact of peer support work on the mental health of peer support specialists. *International Journal of Mental Health Systems* 16, 51. https://doi.org/10.1186/s13033-022-00561-8

Repper, J., Aldridge, B., Gilfoyle, S., Gillard, S., Perkins, R. & Rennison, J. (2013) *Peer Support Workers: Theory and Practice* (Internet). Available at: https://static1.squaresp ace.com/static/65e873c27971d37984653be0/t/668ce21ba54f933596890e57/172050 8956537/5ImROC-Peer-Support-Workers-Theory-and-Practice.pdf (Accessed 27 January 2025).

Robertson, S., Leigh-Phippard, H., Robertson, D., Thomson, A., Casey, J. & Walsh, L.J. (2024) What supports the emotional well-being of peer workers in an NHS mental health service? *Mental Health and Social Inclusion.* https://doi.org/10.1108/MHSI-02-2024-0023

Schon, U.-K. (2010) The power of identification: Peer support in recovery from mental illness. *Scandinavian Journal of Disability Research* 12(2), 83–90. https://doi.org/10.1108/MHSI-02-2024-0023

Shalaby, R.A.H. & Agyapong, V.I.O. (2020) Peer support in mental health: Literature review. *JMIR Mental Health* 7(6), e15572. https://doi.org/10.2196/15572

Simpson, A., Oster, C. & Muir-Cochrane, E. (2017) Liminality in the occupational identity of mental health peer support workers: A qualitative study. *International Journal of Mental Health Nursing* 27(2), 662–671. https://doi.org/10.1111/inm.12351

Slade, M. & Longden, E. (2015) Empirical evidence about recovery and mental health. *BMC Psychiatry* 15, 285. https://doi.org/10.1186/s12888-015-0678-4

Trachtenberg, M., Parsonage, M., Shepherd, G. & Boardman, J. (n.d.) *Peer Support in Mental Health Care: Is It Good Value for Money?* (Internet). Available at: www.researchi ntorecovery.com/files/RRNJuly13_2013_ImROCPeersupport%20workersvalueformo ney.pdf (Accessed 27 January 2025).

Watson, E. & Repper, J. (n.d.) *Peer Support in Mental Health and Social Care Services: Where Are We Now* (Internet). Available at: www.imroc.org/publications/peer-support-in-men tal-health-and-social-care-services-where-are-we-now (Accessed 27 January 2025).

Watts, M. (2012) *Recovery from 'Mental Illness' as a Re-Enchantment with Life: A Narrative Study.* PhD Dissertation, University of Dublin, Trinity College.

Part 4

Policy Relating to Peer Support Work

Chapter 10

Policy Developments in Support of Peer Support Work

10.1 Introduction

For the past few chapters, our central focus has been on the latest research debates on peer support work in mental health. This was an important aspect of the text as it demonstrates the current fluidity of the field and how central issues like that of experiential knowledge or ethical informality are only now arising in the literature. This present chapter represents the only chapter in this text that will have a specific focus on policy. Such discussions are important to showcase the various cultural and indeed political underpinnings of peer support work currently being expressed within related policy documents that are central to the development of mental health services on a national or transnational basis. The chapter begins with Section 10.2 which will explore specifically the Irish policy documents that have led to the implementation and continuous development of peer support work in this jurisdiction. Section 10.3, adds a layer to such discussions by exploring the same through a UK lens followed by Section 10.4 that will look explicitly at American policy development in this area. After this point the text will take its focus off the global north through an examination of Australian mental health policy in Section 10.5 followed by an Asian angle in Section 10.6 which will examine Chinese mental health policy in this area. The chapter will then conclude with a summary of what has been learned in this specific chapter and how this can influence the remainder of this text. This will occur in Section 10.7.

10.2 Mental Health Policy in the Republic of Ireland

Within an Irish context, two policies have been instrumental in advocating for the need for Peer Support Workers within mental health services. The first is '*A Vision for Change: Report on the Expert Group on Mental Health Policy*' (Department of Health, 2006). This document was a catalyst for instrumental change within mental health service provision by advocating for the closure of the traditional asylums of that time and replacing same with community services, in which multi-disciplinary teams form a central component (Norton, 2022). Additionally, the policy began conversations relating to the concept of personal recovery, which later allowed

DOI: 10.4324/9781032717050-14

for a nationwide programme to be established to embed recovery in mental health discourse (Norton and Cullen, 2024). Within '*A Vision for Change*' in Chapter 18 the policy stipulates:

> Within the expanded model of the community mental health team it is proposed to create a new position of mental health support worker. These new workers in the mental health system will provide service users with companionship, friendship and practical support with daily living activities. They will help service users gain access to services and resources such as housing and employment. The new staff may come from a wide range of educational backgrounds with diverse personal experiences and qualifications. Some **may be users, carers,** nursing assistants or retired staff. They should be offered flexible arrangements in terms of working hours to maximise their value to the service user.
>
> (Department of Health, 2006, p.195)

In addition, the policy also noted the implementation of a mental health support worker as a recommendation which policy enforcers must try and achieve. The recommendation states that: '*the position of mental health support worker be established in the mental health system to support service users in achieving independent living and integration in their local community*' (Department of Health, 2006, p. 195, Recommendation 18.24). The above extract from '*A Vision for Change*' and its accompanying recommendation is important for the development of Peer Support Workers as a profession in Irish, statutory services. This is the case as underlined and bolded in the text above is a suggestion that such mental health support workers '… *may be users, carers…*' (p. 195). The use of these specific words in the policy paved the way for the introduction of Peer Support Workers in Irish mental health services as it suggests that such workers can be former service users of the mental health services and/or carers of those utilising these same services (Naughton et al., 2015).

In later years, the Department of Health recognised that more work was required to achieve the optimal service for everyone (Swords and Norton, 2020). As such, on 17 June 2020, the next iteration of '*A Vision for Change*', '*Sharing the Vision: A Mental Health Policy for Everyone*' (Department of Health, 2020) was published. This new policy has 100 recommendations, all of which are necessary to further transform the services by the year 2030 (Department of Health, 2022). Within which the further development on the role of the peer in mental health service provision is noted via recommendation 74 which states:

> *The HSE should continue to develop, fund and periodically evaluate existing and new peer-led/peer-run services provided to people with mental health difficulties across the country.*
>
> (Department of Health, 2020, p. 104)

Most notably, this recommendation advocates for the future development of peer roles across a multitude of mental health support settings. As a result, this recommendation is 1 of 11 that were assigned by the Minister to the now Office of Mental Health Engagement and Recovery (MHER) – an office that was formed by the fusion of the Office of Mental Health Engagement and Advancing Recovery in Ireland – the pilot initiative set up as a result of '*A Vision for Change*' responsible for implementing recovery orientated services in an Irish context (Health Service Executive, 2023). Within an Irish context, peer support work in all its forms remains a strategic priority, not just for MHER but for all services collectively to reach the policy goal of recovery orientation and a mental health service that is truly available for anyone.

10.3 Mental Health Policy in the UK

Irish mental health policy closely aligns with that published in the UK due to a number of factors including the proximity of the two jurisdictions and the colonisation of Ireland by the British until recent years (Cullen and Norton, 2024). Within a UK context, their equivalent to '*Sharing the Vision*' is the '*NHS Mental Health Implementation Plan 2019/20-2023/24*' (National Health Service [NHS], 2019). This policy, which was the successor of '*The Five Year Forward View for Mental Health*' policy (NHS, 2016) and is aimed specifically to make transformative changes in the provision of mental health services through an examination of specific needs for specific populations such as children and young people, crisis services and digital mental health to name just a few (Cullen and Norton, 2024).

Within the '*NHS Mental Health Implementation Plan 2019/20-2023/24*' the focus seems to be on the continuous development of the Peer Support Worker role. This is not surprising given that Peer Support Workers have been implemented in the UK since 2009 (Watson and Repper, n.d.). Within the policy document, it is predicted that the peer support workforce will grow to 150 by the end of last year (2024) (NHS, 2019). These posts have the potential of being in the specialised services as it states:

> *Targeted workforce development for adult eating disorders and complex mental health difficulties associated with a diagnosis of 'personality disorder' will also be undertaken in partnership with HEE including exploring key non-clinical roles, such as peer support workers, and the development of the mental health pharmacist workforce.*

(NHS, 2019, p. 27)

In addition to this, the policy advocates for the involvement of Peer Support Workers within specialist crisis care services including crisis houses/cafés (NHS, 2019). This is similar to that expressed in Ireland's '*Sharing the Vision*' policy under recommendations 24 and 74 (Norton, 2023). Whilst services await a new implementation plan, the NHS released their priorities for 2024/25 in March last year (2024). Although peer support was not highlighted as a priority, it is implied through the wording used including '*...more personalised and joined up care...*'

and '*improve [the] quality of mental health activity [and] outcomes ...*' (NHS Confederation, 2024).

10.4 The USA

Unlike Ireland and the UK, Peer Support Workers[1] have been in place within mental health service provision in the USA since Georgia received Medicaid approval in 1999 to develop the role (Center for Psychiatric Rehabilitation, 2022). As such it is not surprising that the US policy document: '*The State of Mental Health in America*' (Mental Health America, 2024) like that of its UK counterpart the '*NHS Mental Health Implementation Plan 2019/20-2023/24*' also focuses on the future development of the Peer Support Worker role rather than its initial implementation within their state's mental health services. This is evident from the following extract from the 2024 edition of their policy document which states:

> *One of the ways to increase access to mental health providers is to expand the use of peer support specialists. SAMHSA recognizes peer support as an effective, evidence-based practice and peer support specialists as central parts of the treatment team. To further expand the use of peer support specialists there must be an increase in the settings in which they practice, the services they provide, and reimbursement for those services... States can also expand the use of peer support specialists in mental health promotion and early intervention services through the rehabilitative option in their Medicaid plans.*
>
> (Mental Health America, 2024, pp. 29–30)

Again, like that of the UK policy document and to an extent the current Irish policy document, there are calls to expand and specialise peer support work in different areas. In this example, through mental health promotion and early intervention initiatives. Interestingly, the US services are beginning to view peers as imperative for the prevention and pro-active prevention of mental health challenges. Something that has yet to arise within other jurisdictions explored so far.

10.5 Australia

Like that of Ireland, the UK, and the USA, Australian mental health policy also seeks to transform the services, but this time to one that is more proactive rather than reactive (Cullen and Norton, 2024). The Australian policy is known as the '*National Mental Health Policy 2008*' (Commonwealth of Australia, 2009) and is one of the oldest policies to be relevant to the development of peer support work today. Interestingly, unlike those examined before, the Australian mental health policy places peer support work as external to the multi-disciplinary team and indeed the mental health services (Commonwealth of Australia, 2009). Instead, they are situated external to the same, finding a home within non-governmental organisations as outlined in the following extract:

The non-governmental sector provides crucial support to individuals, as well as to carers and families. Non-government sector services include psychiatric disability support services, advocacy services, peer support services, consumer-operated services and programs addressing areas such as living skills, vocational training, accommodation support and respite care.

(Commonwealth of Australia, 2009)

In addition to this, like the policies discussed earlier, the '*National Mental Health Policy 2008*' also advocates for specialisations within the sector that support individuals' mental health. Within the policy, this is noted through the recognition of the need for Peer Support Workers with Aboriginal and Torres Strait Islander ethnic backgrounds (Commonwealth of Australia, 2009). Since the publication of this policy, in 2024, the first official guidelines to support the introduction of Aboriginal and Torres Strait Islander peer workers have been produced with a unique set of roles and functions necessary to engage effectively and compassionately with this indigenous community (Lee et al., 2024).

10.6 China

The final jurisdiction in which we will explore mental health policy that is conducive to peer support work comes not from the global north or Australia but instead is situated in Asia in a country which has one of the largest populations in the entire world. China was identified as a jurisdiction worth exploring due to the increasing literature base arising from this jurisdiction in regard to peer support work in mental health. See for example Tse et al. (2013), Chen et al. (2024) and Fan et al. (2024). In China, the policy by which mental health services operate is the '*National Mental Health Work Plan (2015–2020)*', translated into English by Xiong and Phillips (2016). Unfortunately, despite the developments within the Chinese peer-reviewed literature to date, mental health policy in this jurisdiction has yet to come to standards set by the peer-reviewed literature in this region. The policy is written with a biomedical lens using phrases like '*mental illness*' and focussed primarily on increasing psychiatrists rather than other multi-disciplinary team professionals (Xiong and Phillips, 2016).

10.7 Concluding Remarks

In summary, this chapter focussed on developments within policy that have led to the rise and continuous development of peer support work within five jurisdictions (Ireland, UK, USA, Australia and China) chosen due to their proliferation in intellectual thought around such work. What is evident within such policy documents is that, for the most part, the peer initiative has been implemented successfully within mental health discourse. As a result, most policies – with the exception of China's – focus on the development of peer services through specialisms targeting various marginalised populations as well as various types of disorders – like personality disorders or eating disorders – or at specific points in the service user journey – such as crisis care. As such, from a policy perspective, peer support has been successful in its implementation and now, in current discourse, is time to specialise peers in various aspects of care. With this in mind, the following three chapters will explore certain levels of peer support specialisms that have emerged throughout the past few years. This will begin, in the following pages, firstly through a critical examination of family peer support work, which is presented in the next chapter.

Note

1 In the United States of America, Peer Support Workers are known as Certified Peer Specialists.

References

Center for Psychiatric Rehabilitation (2022) *The Peer Support Specialist Workforce: Where Have We Been and Where Are We Going?* (Internet). Available at: https://cpr.bu.edu/blog-the-peer-support-workforce/ (Accessed 29 January 2025).

Chen, X., Qin, S., Sheehan, L., Ma, Z., Spicknall, V. & Fan, Y. (2024) A feasibility evaluation of a peer support intervention for social participation in China. *Journal of Public Mental Health* 23(3), 217–228. https://doi.org/10.1108/JPMH-01-2024-0011

Commonwealth of Australia (2009) *National Mental Health Policy 2008* (Internet). Available at: www.health.gov.au/sites/default/files/documents/2020/11/national-mental-health-policy-2008.pdf, (Accessed 29 January 2025).

Cullen, O.J. & Norton, M.J. (2024) Mental health, addiction and dual diagnoses: National and international policy context. In *Different Diagnoses, Similar Experiences: Narratives of Mental Health, Addiction Recovery and Dual Diagnosis* (Norton, M.J. & Cullen, O.J. eds.). Emerald Publishing Limited, Leeds, pp. 19–33.

Department of Health (2006) *A Vision for Change: Report of the Expert Group on Mental Health Policy* (Internet). Available at: www.hse.ie/eng/services/publications/mentalhealth/mental-health---a-vision-for-change.pdf, (Accessed 28 January 2025).

Department of Health (2020) *Sharing the Vision: A Mental Health Policy for Everyone* (Internet). Available at: www.lenus.ie/bitstream/handle/10147/633416/76770_b142b216-f2ca-48e6-a551-79c208f1a247%281%29.pdf?sequence=1&isAllowed=y (Accessed 29 January 2025).

Department of Health (2022) *Implementation Plan 2022–2024: Sharing the Vision: A Mental Health Policy for Everyone* (Internet). Available at: https://assets.gov.ie/static/documents/sharing-the-vision-implementation-plan-2022-2024.pdf (Accessed 29 January 2025).

Fan, Y., Liu, X. & Li, C. (2024) Experiences of naturally occurring peer support among people using psychiatric day-care in China: An interpretative phenomenological approach. *Frontiers in Psychiatry* 15, 1349778. https://doi.org/10.3389/fpsyt.2024.1349778

Health Service Executive (2023) *Strategic Plan 2023–2026: Engaged in Recovery* (Internet). Available at: www.hse.ie/eng/services/list/4/mental-health-services/mental-health-engagement-and-recovery/mher-strategic-plan-engaged-in-recovery.pdf (Accessed 29 January 2025).

Lee, T., Mckenna, R., Morseau, G., Bacon, A., Baguley, K., Cowdrey-Fong, S., Bertakis, A., Shorey, T., Smith, T., Mckenna, V., Kitchener, E. & Meteoro, N. (2024) *Aboriginal and Torres Strait Islander Lived Experience-Led Peer Workforce Guide: A Learning*

Tool for All Peer Workforces and Organisations (Internet). Available at: www.mhc. wa.gov.au/media/5021/mhc24-63121-v7-ilec-blackdog-aboriginal-lived-experience-peer-led-workforce-guide-v11-july-2024-final-version-attachment-1.pdf (Accessed 29 January 2025).

Mental Health America (2024) *The State of Mental Health in America: 2024 Edition* (Internet). Available at: https://mhanational.org/sites/default/files/2024-State-of-Mental-Health-in-America-Report.pdf (Accessed 29 January 2025).

National Health Service (NHS) (2016) *The Five Year Forward View for Mental Health* (Internet). Available at: www.england.nhs.uk/wp-content/uploads/2016/02/Mental-Hea lth-Taskforce-FYFV-final.pdf (Accessed 29 January 2025).

National Health Service (NHS) (2019) *NHS Mental Health Implementation Plan 2019/ 20-2023/24* (Internet). Available at: www.longtermplan.nhs.uk/wp-content/uploads/ 2019/07/nhs-mental-health-implementation-plan-2019-20-2023-24.pdf (Accessed 29 January 2025).

Naughton, L., Collins, P. & Ryan, M. (2015) *Peer Support Workers: A Guidance Paper* (Internet). Available at: www.lenus.ie/bitstream/handle/10147/576059/PeerSupportWo rkersAGuidancePaper.pdf?sequence=6 (Accessed 28 January 2025).

NHS Confederation (2024) *2024/25 NHS Priorities and Operational Planning Guidance: What you Need to Know* (Internet). Available at: www.nhsconfed.org/publi cations/202425-nhs-priorities-and-operational-planning-guidance#:~:text=NHSE's%20 overall%20aim%20in%202024,line%20with%20the%20Core20PLUS5%20approach (Accessed 29 January 2025).

Norton, M. (2022) *Co-Production in Mental Health: Implementing Policy into Practice.* Routledge, Oxon.

Norton, M.J. (2023) Mental health peer-led cafés – A complimentary approach to traditional crisis care: A protocol for a systematic scoping review. *Psychiatry International* 4, 370–379. https://doi.org/10.3390/psychiatryint404033

Norton, M.J. & Cullen, O.J. (2024) Contextual and personal introduction to the text. In *Different Diagnoses, Similar Experiences: Narratives of Mental Health, Addiction Recovery and Dual Diagnosis* (Norton, M.J. & Cullen, O.J. eds.). Emerald Publishing Limited, Leeds, pp. 3–18.

Swords, C. & Norton, M.J. (2020) Is sharing really caring? A vision or an aspiration? Ireland's new mental health policy 2020. *Irish Journal of Psychological Medicine.* https:// doi.org/10.1017/ipm.2020.118

Tse, S., Tsoi, E.W.S., Wong, S., Kan, A. & Kwok, C.F.-Y. (2013) Training of mental health peer support workers in a non-western high-income city: Preliminary evaluation and experience. *International Journal of Social Psychiatry* 60(3), 211–218. https://doi.org/ 10.1177/0020764013481427

Watson, E. & Repper, J. (n.d.) *Peer Support in Mental Health and Social Care Services: Where Are We Now?* (Internet). Available at: www.imroc.org/publications/peer-support-in-men tal-health-and-social-care-services-where-are-we-now (Accessed 29 January 2025).

Xiong, W. & Phillips, M.R. (2016) Translated and annotated version of the 2015–2020 national mental health work plan of the People's Republic of China. *Shanghai Archives of Psychiatry* 28(1), 4–17. https://doi.org/10.11919/j.issn.1002-0829.216012

Part 5

The Practice of Peer Support Work

Chapter 11

Family Peer Support Work

Case Study Contributor:

Matthew Jackman

11.1 Introduction

Up to this point, we have explored much of the discourse relating to peer support work in mental health. This has been from a theory, research and policy perspective. This present chapter marks the first of three chapters that will focus on the practice of peer support work. This includes critical discussions on peer support specialisms and also discussion relating to current practices as noted within the nine case studies collected for this text (Case Study 9 will be presented in this chapter). We begin discussions on the practice of peer support work in this chapter by examining the specialist role of the Family Peer Support Worker and how they are similar but distinctly different to their service user peer counterparts. We begin with Section 11.2 which will examine the relatively new concept of family recovery within mental health discourse. This is followed by an exploration into the definition and role of the Family Peer Support Worker in Section 11.3. Section 11.4 describes the unique referral process for those seeking to engage with a family peer – utilising the Irish referral process as an example. Section 11.5 then supports the conclusion of this exploration by providing a list of recommendations and resources for those wishing to embed Family Peer Support Workers in their service. Finally, Section 11.6 will conclude the chapter by summarising the key learnings to be taken from this critical exploration.

11.2 Family Recovery in Mental Health

The recognition that family members of individuals with mental health challenges have their own unique needs that need to be addressed in unison with the individual suffering from a mental health challenge is a relatively new development within the mental health discourse. This has led to a new typology of recovery, known as family recovery which is still growing empirically today (Norton and Cullen, 2024). In an Irish context, family recovery is defined as:

DOI: 10.4324/9781032717050-16

re-establishing our roles, goals, ambitions, and lives, it's about learning to maintain our wellbeing and resilience so that we can continue to support our family members/friend's recovery.

(Office of Mental Health Engagement and Recovery,
Mental Health Ireland and REFOCUS, 2018, p. 1)

This definition recognises that the individual family member has a life of their own to live and explore and that one needs to ensure they practice self-care even when supporting a loved one with a mental illness. Again, within an Irish context, this idea was first recognised when the then Advancing Recovery in Ireland (ARI) co-produced the '*Family Recovery Guidance Document 2018-2020*' (Health Service Executive, 2018) to coincide with the publication of the first iteration of '*A National Framework for Recovery in Mental Health 2018–2020*' (Health Service Executive, 2017). Within this co-produced guidance document, it recognises that when a member of the family has a mental health challenge, the whole family requires support to engage in their own recovery journey (Health Service Executive, 2018). However, at this time, familial lived experiences were not recognised. In fact, it was a number of years later, when the current '*A National Framework for Recovery in Mental Health 2024–2028*' was published in 2024 that familial lived experiences were recognised. In this framework, principle one was revised to just state '*the centrality of lived experience*' (Health Service Executive, 2024). This is an important development as simply removing service users from principle one allows for the recognition of familial lived experience at a strategic, policy level within mental health discourse.

Although research into familial lived experiences and family recovery are in their infancy, a 2021 systematic review conducted by Norton and Cuskelly, identified a number of enablers of family recovery – in other words, the elements that support family recovery in mental health. Here, they identified written information, access to information and support as examples of such family recovery enablers (Norton and Cuskelly, 2021). In addition, due to the nature of the original review conducted by Norton and Cuskelly, a protocol for a scoping review was subsequently developed and published by Cuskelly et al. (2022) to state the authors' intentions to explore family recovery enablers further through a scoping review to examine the breadth of literature into the concept. This review is currently underway and it is hoped it will be published in mid-2025. Additionally, in conjunction with developments relating to family recovery and familial lived experience, there are now calls for services to engage in a whole-family approach to mental health service provision (Maynooth University, 2024). This involves addressing the needs of families in parallel to that of the mental health service user (Maynooth University, 2024). However, each of these concepts is in its infancy, with further empirical studies required to develop a firm evidence base for family-orientated practices within mental health service provision both in Ireland and internationally.

11.3 Family Peer Support Work

Like that of peer support work, family peer support is also another difficult term to define. However, for the purposes of this text, we will define family peer support work as per noted by Orygen (n.d.). Here, family peer support work is defined as a reciprocal relationship that involves an individual with lived experiences of caring for a loved one with mental health challenges supporting another family/family member who is at an earlier phase of their own recovery journey (Orygen, n.d.). This definition suggests that like service users, family members have their own lived experience that differentiates from service user's lived experience due to the positionality of the host towards the experience itself.

Additionally, like that of the service user Peer Support Worker, Family Peer Support Workers also have a set of core values. These include inclusivity, respect, reciprocity and mutuality (Pachowicz and Goffe, 2024). Although similar to that of the service user peer, the mechanism by which inclusivity, respect, reciprocity and mutuality are established and maintained differ due to the positionality of the person to the distress experienced by their loved one. Indeed, the fact that family members have little interaction with actors diminishes their sense of autonomy, power and self-agency, the mechanism of creating informality is shorter and easier to maintain over time as these individuals are often met external to the traditional mental health system. What helps in this venture is that such family peers are external to traditional mental health systems which inadvertently does not require them to break down as many hierarchical barriers as that is required when dealing with both service users and Peer Support Workers who are very much internal within mental health service provision.

Despite these differences in positionality and functionality, Family Peer Support Workers are still required to undergo specialised training to utilise their experiences effectively to support individual family members who are in an earlier phase of recovery (Center of Innovation for Behavioural Health and Wellbeing, 2023; The Housing Agency, 2024). Once qualified and hired by a mental health service, they are responsible for carrying out their role in compliance with the associated job specifications. In Appendix, I provide an example of a template job specification for family peers. In addition, the National Health Service (NHS) in the UK also provides a figure depicting the various roles and responsibilities of the Peer Support Worker (Figure 11.1) (NHS Health Education England, 2020).

Pachowicz and Goffe (2024) in a recent report on Family Peer Support Workers noted that these competencies, noted in Figure 11.1 are also applicable to that of the family peer. However, there is much debate in practice currently as to the differences and similarities between the service user and family Peer Support Worker roles. In Case Study 9, Matthew brings us through what it is like working as a peer and then as a family peer within a forensic mental health service in Australia in which they note the competing and comparing roles of being a peer and a family peer.

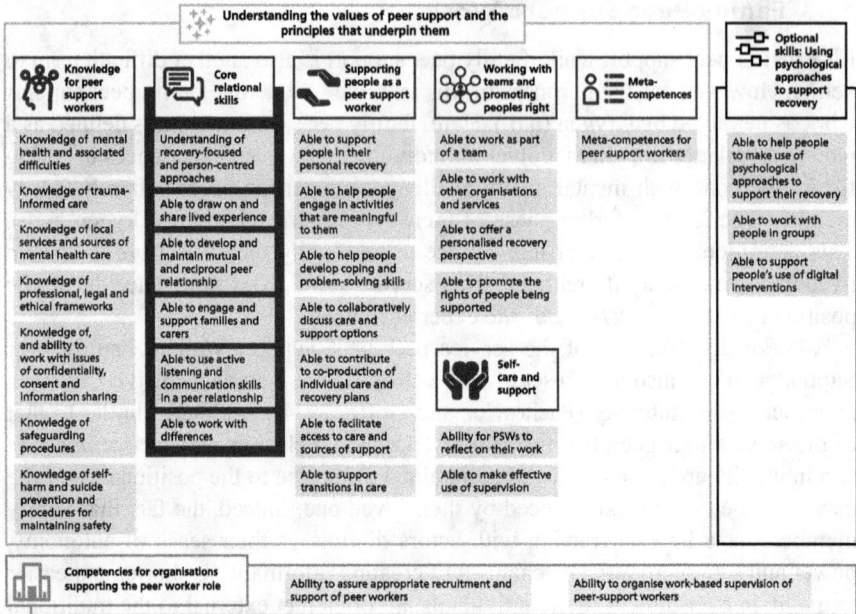

Figure 11.1 Competency Map of Mental Health Peer and Family Peer Support Workers.

Case Study 9   Consumer and Carer Leadership and Participation in Forensic Mental HealthPeer Work in a Risk Aversive Culture

Matthew Jackman

How I Came to Peer Work, as a Young Carer, Social Work Student, and Person with Lived Experience

I was a naïve social work student who had come to studying the discipline as primarily a young carer, who had experienced my own mental health difficulties particularly because of my mother's suicide, ongoing child abuse and neglect, and family violence in the home until my mid teenage years. My fathers' partners were often the source of violence, and his neglect to keep a home and financial stability meant disruption in other areas. All I knew was how to care for other people, from my mother to my younger siblings, to parenting my own father and protecting everyone from his partners abuse often induced by substances and underlying mental health issues. I experienced acute suicidal thoughts at the age of 19 and attempted suicide but told no one about it. I moved home to a regional area, with no friends, in a home my father could afford as a single parent. As a young queer person who was not out at the time, I did not even understand I had mental health issues. They weren't discussed, much like gender and sexuality in the 2000s, especially in a large multicultural low socio-economic school, so I had little literacy and family capacity, and resilience to support myself and find this thing we call 'recovery' now. I often advocated for my siblings who in my early 20s were in and out of psychiatric hospitals with issues around substances and what psychiatry labelled schizophrenia.

Once again, thrust into over-parentified child and now young adult, I neglected my own mental health issues, which were always present and emerged from complex trauma, grief and loss, abandonment from my mother's parents after her suicide, and ongoing social issues such as moving house, my father's unstable employment and finances resulting in material deprivation, and homophobia, which kept me in the closet for a few more years. It was fear of being myself, that lead to my first suicide attempt, nothing biomedical, just a society not accepting me for who I am, including my father, who told me '*Gay people are diseased*' when I was aged 15. I did not come out for another five years as a result, and almost lost my life. I tell part of my story, as this contextualises coming to study social work and encountering peer work, namely consumer work, in Australia, where we use consumer perspectives developed from the consumer movements collective knowledge to inform how we support our peers.

From Social Work Training to Entering Peer Work Leadership in Forensic Mental Health: An Introduction to Consumer Consultancy 'systemic advocacy'

It was my final social work placement in forensic mental health where I would meet the consumer consultant team, led by an incredible woman, who ended up being my entry into the consumer movement world, and my passion for systemic advocacy. My placement involved supporting consumer consultants, as by nature there were periods were they were distressed and/or requiring a break, and I would support them given the known intersecting lived experience I had by the social work manager of the forensic hospital, who happened to be a massive fan of my work. I volunteered to come in on the weekend to support the annual carers day with the family consultant, who supported the families and carers to meet, as they had their own stories of trauma, grief and loss, and dually stigmatised around issues of mental health and criminal justice.

Upon graduation, I was employed the following week by the forensic hospital to work in the consumer consultant team. In this role, I was nourished and mentored by a senior consumer consultant who was highly regarded in the Australian consumer movement particularly around her work with women and gendered services. Like me, she was queer, and a feminist and I think this intersectionality and shared layering of oppression brought us to the work in the broader consumer, psychiatric survivor, users and as users of psychiatry, and Mad movement. I was fortunate to represent consumers by attending community meetings each morning and providing messages to consumers of activities for participation, such as artwork, recovery planning, feedback surveys and other ways for consumers to participate in paid capacities to improve the forensic hospital systemically. Some key issues raised included patients, which they preferred to be named in a forensic setting to acknowledge the mental illness component of what had occurred in the context of a not guilty by reasons of mental impairment defence, such as waters coolers in each unit, and more friendly and warm hospital wards. I would help to cofacilitate consumer advisory groups where one patient from each unit would raise feedback on behalf of consumers on their unit and bring them to the monthly 'CAG', which was a consumer advisory group where consumer representatives from each unit who would bring issues from acute issues, to rehabilitation, to women's unit issues to discuss key issues on behalf of their forensic units with the consumer consultants where we would invite key leaders in the organisation to attend, dialogue and present their own agenda for co-production such as the inpatient director, nursing and allied health managers, and sometimes we would have external visitors presenting on issues around human rights such as the independent mental health advocacy service where patients were allocated an opt in advocate when placed on a forensic order.

Furthermore, another group we would co-facilitate with other patients, would be the patient recovery group, where we would work together on recovery plans for nurses to implement with the care team in partnership with the patients, to see their personal goals, wishes, aspirations, and dreams, alongside 'clinical' also known as medical and symptom remission recovery goals which were often about risk management, forensic issues, and leave restrictions based on a system of reward and punishment. I thoroughly enjoyed following up in a peer support capacity with patients, in discussing what issues that were most important to them, as this was their home, often for average eight to ten years, and many were institutionalised and even frightened to go back into community. The consumer consultant team would work particularly close with the social work and occupational therapy teams as a result, to assist with both participation within the hospital, such as vocational needs and skills, addressing cultural needs and issues, spiritual needs and issues, and basic human rights around dignity of risk and an overall risk aversive culture based on fear mongering and media portrayals of '*absconded*' patients being violent, and dangerous.

The patients whom I worked alongside to support as people, were some of the most kind, thoughtful, generous, insightful and intelligent human beings I had ever met. I am speaking about a time in my life, ten years prior to writing this contribution. Consequently, some of the most rewarding moments have come from bumping into these folk who have been discharged or nearing discharge from the forensic hospital on overnight community leave in my own community as two citizens, where if they engage with me, which they always do, wish them a warm welcome and tell them how proud I am. I always ask how they're finding the new environment and talk about community events. It's always a brief, but meaningful conversation, and I can sense they feel a difference was made in their life during our past history working together, and then in my acceptance and embracing in the community.

A large part of the role was ensuring we met consumer participation standards for the statewide health audit, where consumer information and education was paramount. We would often communicate messages from executive to consumers through both the 'CAG' and regular inpatient unit meetings, but also relay messages as we would bump into people walking around the high secure forensic hospital setting. The hospital was 116 beds at the time and has continued to triple in the proceeding ten years, calling into question issues around re-institutionalisation of the asylum era and incarcerating mental health as was done during the poor law and workhouse period. This current forensic mental health trend calls for abolition and Mad studies to offer unique approaches that are peer driven and lead, and call for ecosystemic change that address both social, structural and commercial determinants in public health such as transformative reform in housing, employment, education and social welfare.

From Consumer Consultancy to Carer Consultancy: An Introduction to Peer Work in Family/Carer Roles in Forensic Mental Health

I digress, as I return to speaking about the consumer consultant role where I started to work with families and carers, and bridge a historic divide between the consumer and family/carer perspective, mostly due to individual differences and personalities, but there was also a history of the family/carer perspective representing human rights restrictions on their loved ones and further risk aversion, which I had compassion for as a sibling and child carer of people where there was harm associated with mental health crises at times in their life, and at times in my own, when experiencing what psychiatry has now labelled bipolar, or my preferred more descriptive term '*manic depressive*'. I wouldn't want to be around a manic irritable me either! Consumer perspectives can be distinguished uniquely from an individual consumer's views. Consumer perspective is a collective theoretical approach, or rather, a discipline borne out of a socio-political movement whereas consumers' views are individual and contextual (Epstein and Shaw, 1997). There is no consensus about what the word consumer means, as certain issues have been identified:

- The language is contested as many consumers dislike the term, believing it to have been adopted by policymakers to appear inclusive. Some believe it does not adequately represent their relationships with clinicians
- The language is contextual, as some people choose to use the word 'consumer' when engaged in advocacy or activism, however, others choose to use the word 'patient' when in hospital. Some prefer terms like 'mad' or 'survivor' in other contexts.
- The language varies internationally: outside of Australia, such terms as 'user' or 'survivor' may be more common (Our Community, 2023).

In my roles, it was vital to have consumer perspective supervision to ensure that I was not further isolated from the underpinning values of my work, especially while working in environments that were pathologising and stigmatising. Supervision is designed to create a space that fosters autonomy, strengths, initiative and creativity .

As I transitioned from the consumer consultant team to the carer consultant team, there was additional opportunity to undertake peer support, and I went and trained in intentional peer support when first introduced to Australia back in 2016. The carer consultant was retiring, and the social work manager had requested I take on the role in transition planning at half her capacity, so I could work alongside another carer who had a different type of carer experience, as now most carers engaging were elderly mothers, and/ or older siblings as the demographic of patients was approximately of middle age. As a carer consultant, I advocated for the needs of families, carers and supporters – both directly and systematically, with the aim of improving the culture and quality of mental health services and the quality of care. Personally, working as a carer consultant has served as a method of activism; within the mental health sector, an increase in activism served to improve services and to increase the consumer and carer voice.

Peer Work, Lateral Violence, and Bullying: Just because You're 'peers', Doesn't Mean You Are 'peers'

The outgoing carer consultant clashed with my new ideas and more progressive and inclusive approach to work more collaboratively with the consumer consultant team I had been in for a few years. I trialled working as a social worker briefly in the women's forensic inpatient unit, and then in prison based counselling and the suicide prevention area of the prisons, and found the experience disheartening, never to return to the realities of social work in practice, which was oppressed and the oppressor within a carceral system designed to entrench and punish those with mental health issues, than promote personal recovery, transformative healing and offer post release support. Social work to me, represented idealism, caught in a system of oppression, and dragged into the mud, with little collectivising, and even less hope as a critical discipline.

Because of the personal clash with my fellow carer consultant, she went around telling other carers she worked with, my future peers I was supposed to support didn't like me, effectively sabotaging the role I was taking over, and I only found this out when a nursing unit manager told me she was bullying me behind my back. This escalated to human resources, and I had a major complex trauma response. At the time I was also working part time in general mental health leading the services first peer work team, which I had to discontinue a few months in, resulting in losing my car I had purchased with the role, and tens of thousands of dollars in debt. I went inward, turning to my old friend and trauma strategy; avoidance, and had major self-doubt and imposter syndrome. I was expected to support families and carers in both peer support and consultancy/systemic advocacy in 10 hours per week across a statewide forensic mental health hospital, community forensic mental health service, and mental health units in three prisons.

I was overwhelmed, dealing with severe bullying, and a serious case of imposter syndrome leading to suicidal thoughts particularly when losing my senior peer work role, losing my car, and losing my professional identity as someone who was a leader and expert in their area of peer leadership practice. Months went by and I began to enter a deep depression, leaving work for days on end, and crying in the car to work on the phone to my father. I couldn't handle the work any longer, and one day attempted to take my life. This resulted in my own engagement with the psychiatric public health system, and from the few months of institutionalisation, I had what I think was a medication induced mania that led to several more periods of depression and mania (Figure 11.2).

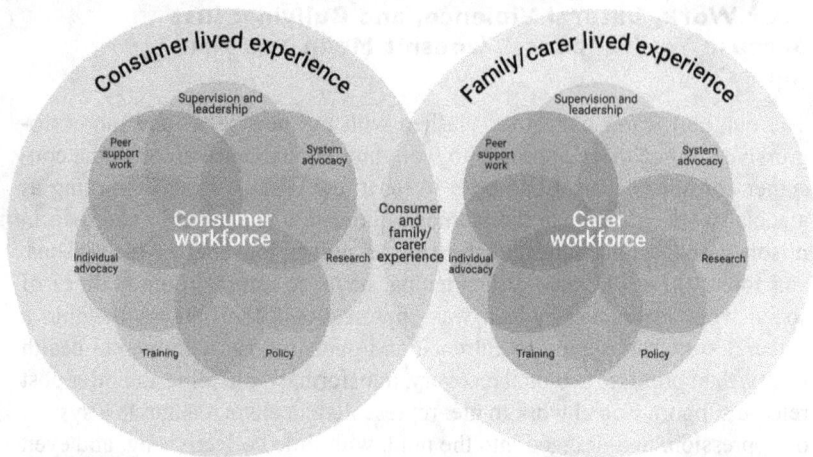

Figure 11.2 Consumer and Family and Carer Lived Experience Work.

The Culmination of Lived, Learnt and Laboured Experience Led to International Mad Activism and Mad Studies

My early experiences of peer work and peer leadership roles, alongside my experiences of being a young carer, living in poverty, being a survivor of trauma, and then a survivor of the psychiatric system, led to an impassioned activist in the Mad pride space. Ironically, I view my experiences very differently to that of my peers in the forensic hospital, as I don't view myself as having an illness, but of responses to trauma, neurodivergence and see my Madness as a source of wisdom. What we do agree on is the basic human rights, dignity, personal recovery and social justice, but that is a story for another day. I often think about the strength and courage of the consumer consultant who taught me the ways, and much like Star Wars, which we both shared a love of, she was the force, and she showed me the light to get through the dark side.

11.4 The Referral Process for Family Peer Support Work: An Irish Context

As noted in Matthew's case study, there are subtle differences between service user Peer Support Workers and their family peer counterparts. Additionally, as evident in Matthew's case study, when one begins to practice traditional peer work on a family peer role, then issues can arise, particularly when dealing with staff who feel that one should practice in a certain way. Within an Irish service, Family Peer Support Workers are mainly based within the community and are separate from the multi-disciplinary team. In other words, family peers sit external to the mental health services but are employed by the service and supervised/line managed by social workers who sit on a multi-disciplinary team. This impacts the family peer in a number of ways including their relationship with traditional service providers, their ability to provide support to families in distress and also in the way family members are referred to their service. Within an Irish context, we have developed in conjunction with the Office of Mental Health Engagement and Recovery (MHER), social work and family peers in a referral pathway that is unique to this role (Figure 11.3). This referral process is now presented as an exemplar for other jurisdictions as to how such family peers work within mental health service provision.

Due to the family peer's distance from the traditional multi-disciplinary team, they can accept referrals from more than one source. Such referral mechanisms include self-referral, referral from community-based organisations like a family resource centre or equivalent and from the community mental health team themselves – usually carried out through the family peer's supervisor/line manager or from their service user peer colleagues. **Please note that this list is non-exhaustive.** Once a referral is received, a screening process occurs to see if the referral is eligible for family peer support input or not. This screening process occurs with the

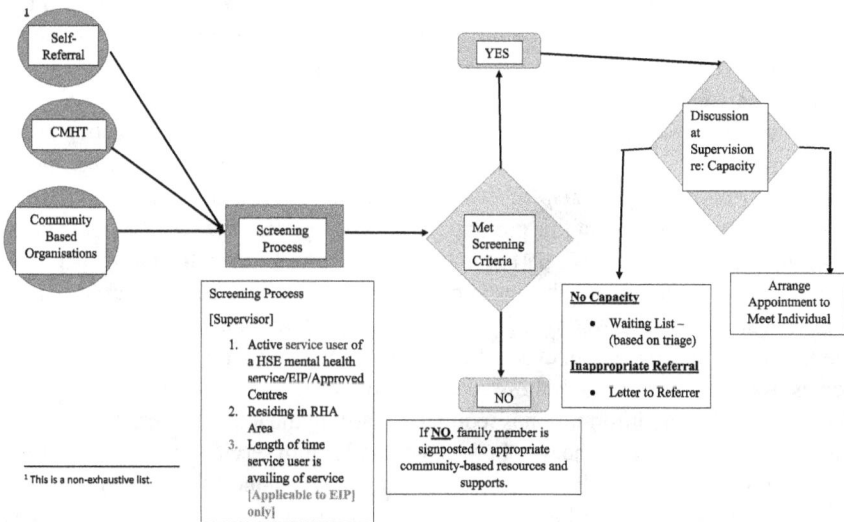

Figure 11.3 Family Peer Support Worker Referral Pathway Process Map.

family peer supervisor during supervision and involves the referral meeting three compulsory criteria:

1. The client has a family member who is currently under the care of the mental health services.
2. The client resides in the same RHA[1] as the family peer.
3. The length of time the client's family member has been availing of the service – **only applicable to those under an early intervention in the psychosis team**. *

If the criteria are not met, the family member is signposted to appropriate community-based resources and supports. If the above criteria are met, a discussion is had as to whether the family peer has the capacity to take on this client. If there is no capacity, the client is placed on a waiting list. If the referral is an inappropriate referral, then a letter is made to the referrer outlining the rationale for not assigning a family peer to this case at this time. If the family peer has the capacity to take on this client, then they are directed to make an initial appointment to meet the client and assess their needs for family peer support work.

11.5 Recommendations and Resources to Advance Family Peer Support Work in Mental Health Discourse

According to Reynolds (2018), the literature base relating to family peer support work is sparse. In 2024, a comprehensive literature review conducted by Pachowicz and Goffe (2024) on behalf of the Office of MHER confirmed such paucity and resulted in the co-creation of 12 core recommendations to support the future progression of family peer support work. These recommendations are presented in Table 11.1.

If implemented correctly, these 12 recommendations would see a dramatic change in how mental health services are delivered. An example of this is an action from recommendation ten which stipulates: '*explore the possibility of integrating family peers into existing multi-disciplinary teams*' (Pachowicz and Goffe, 2024, p. 10). If a service was to implement this particular recommendation, the service would have to acknowledge the family as part of the treatment team and that the family peer has something of value to give that extends beyond what a service user Peer Support Worker can do. It also would suggest that the family member is entitled to know the status of their loved one, even when this is damaging to the service users themselves. As such, even though these recommendations from the literature are gratefully received, more information is required regarding the impact of employing such mechanisms will have on the way in which mental health service provision operates.

Within Irish mental health services, the Family Peer Support Workers in situ have developed a website to further support their integration into mental health services (Family Peer Support Service n.d.a).[2] This resource (link in footnote) is an invaluable resource for families trying to understand their loved one's mental health challenges, as well as information that they can use to support their own well-being. In addition, the Office of MHER, the office responsible for the development of peer

Table 11.1 Recommendations for the Future Progression of Family Peer Support Work Here

No.	Recommendation	Action
1	Place Family Peer Support Workers and family members at the lead of all future developments in family peer support work.	Co-produce Family Peer Support Worker's role description, requirements and other relevant documentation with family members and family peers.
		Co-produce and co-deliver Family Peer Support Worker training with family peers and family members.
		Support and find research led by family members into family peer support
2	Co-produce a set of core values for Family Peer Support Workers.	Any co-produced core values should be specific to Family Peer Support Workers.
		Core values should be reviewed annually so that revisions and changes can be made if necessary.
3	Clearly define the aims of the work conducted by Family Peer Support Workers in mental health services.	Any defined aims should be specific to Family Peer Support Workers.
		Any defined aims must align with the values and principles of family peer support work.
		Any defined aims should be flexible enough as to not compromise the client-led nature of family peer support work.
4	Enhance the accessibility of family peer support work.	Avoid restricting access to the family peer to specific relatives.
		Implement family peer support in a range of modes and settings.
		Explore the possibility of drop-in sessions within acute services, primary care and day hospitals.
		Expand reach to all family members of people experiencing mental health difficulties, not just to those who are family members of clients attending mental health services.
		Establish an online, open repository for family member resources.

(Continued)

Table 11.1 (Continued)

No.	Recommendation	Action
5	Co-produce a core competency framework for Family Peer Support Workers in the mental health services.	Such core competency frameworks should be specific to Family Peer Support Workers.
		These core competencies should reflect the values and principles of family peer support work.
		The core competencies should be reviewed annually.
6	Co-produce standardised guidelines for the recruitment of Family Peer Support Workers within mental health services.	All recruitment material for Family Peer Support Workers should be co-produced with family peers and family members.
		Such material should define the roles and responsibilities of Family Peer Support Workers.
		Family Peer Support Workers should be involved in the recruitment of new family peers.
		Ensure that prospective Family Peer Support Workers have a minimum level of education to work in the role – including appropriate literacy and numeracy assessments.
7	Develop accessible training programmes and certification mechanisms for Family Peer Support Workers, led by family members and existing Family Peer Support Workers.	Co-produce introductory and ongoing training for family peers.
		All co-produced training for family peers should reflect the core competencies discussed in recommendation 5.
		Minimise training costs by providing scholarships, grants and subsidies for family peers who want to enhance their education in line with their respective duties as a Family Peer Support Worker.

8	Explore the possibility of recruiting specialised Family Peer Support Workers with specific lived experience or from specific backgrounds or communities.	Establish if there is a need for specialised family peers.
		Ensure that any recruitment of specialised family peers is culturally appropriate and led by members of the relevant communities.
9	Provide Family Peer Support Workers with regular, appropriate supervision.	Employ experienced family peers to supervise junior colleagues.
		Ensure protective time so that family peers can avail of appropriate supervision.
		Ensure adequate training and support for family peer supervisors.
10	Support the integration of Family Peer Support Workers into mental health services by actively addressing unhelpful attitudes and cultural factors.	Provide co-produced training on family peer support work for existing staff within the mental health services.
		Continue to support the meaningful inclusion of the voice of service users and their families into service design, delivery and evaluation.
		Explore the possibility of integrating family peers into existing multi-disciplinary teams.
11	Standardise data collection across all family peer support work services.	Record the number, type and duration of Family Peer Support Worker's contact with clients.
		Collect and record demographic data of those family peers work with.
		Explore the possibility co-creating a validated, quantitative measurement tool for family peer support work services.
		Conduct regular nationwide surveys on the family peer support workforce to collect demographic characteristics, experiences and needs.
12	Ensure that Family Peer Support Workers employed in the mental health services are adequately supported.	Provide flexible working arrangements for the Family Peer Support Worker.
		In addition to the employee assistance programme, offer Family Peer Support Workers confidential, one-on-one psychological and/or counselling support.
		Establish a nationwide Family Peer Support Workers network.

Source: Pachowicz and Goffe (2024).

support within an Irish context have also produced a video that is freely available on YouTube, which is used to introduce family peer support work to anyone interested in the same (link in footnote) (Family Peer Support Service, n.d.b).[3]

11.6 Concluding Remarks

This chapter was the first of three to discuss the practice of peer support work. In this particular chapter, we explored the specialist role of family peer support work. Within this we explored the importance of family recovery and how each individual family member has their own unique recovery journey to follow when a loved one is diagnosed and undergoes a mental health challenge. We also explored the referral pathway for family peer support, utilising the Irish referral pathway as an example. Finally, we explored recommendations from a recent literature review regarding the future development of family peer support work and we also identified resources, specific to an Irish context to demonstrate to other jurisdictions how an area can create something similar for their own family peer support service context. What follows in Chapter 12 is an exploration of the various specialisms of peer support work already noted within the academic and grey literature.

Notes

1   Regional Health Area.
2   https://familypeersupport.ie/
3   www.youtube.com/watch?v=4sIlfHDiqcw

References

Center of Innovation for Behavioural Health and Wellbeing (2023) *Family Peer Support* (Internet). Available at: https://centerofinnovationnm.org/family-peer-support/ (Accessed 30 January 2025).

Cuskelly, K., Norton, M.J. & Delaney, G. (2022) Examining the existing knowledge base for enablers of family recovery in mental health: A protocol for a scoping review of national and international literature. *BMJ Open* 12, e066484. https://doi.org/10.1136/bmjopen-2022-066484

Epstein, M. & Shaw, J. (1997). *Developing Effective Consumer Participation in Mental Health Services: The Report of the Lemon Tree Learning Project.* Victorian Mental Illness Awareness Council, Australia.

Family Peer Support Service (n.d.a) *A New Approach to Family Mental Health Recovery in Ireland* (Internet). Available at: https://familypeersupport.ie/ (Accessed 03 February 2025).

Family Peer Support Service (n.d.b) *A Message from Family Peer Support Workers* (Internet). Available at: https://familypeersupport.ie/a-message-from-family-peer-support-workers (Accessed 03 February 2025).

Health Service Executive (2017) *A National Framework for Recovery in Mental Health 2018–2020: A National Framework for Mental Health Service Providers to Support the*

Delivery of a Quality, Person-Centred Service. Advancing Recovery in Ireland, Dublin, Ireland.

Health Service Executive (2018) *Family Recovery Guidance Document 2018–2020: Supporting 'A National Framework for Recovery in Mental Health 2018–2020'* (Internet). Available at: www.hse.ie/eng/services/list/4/mentalhealth-services/advancing recoveryireland/national-framework-for-recovery-in-mental-health/family-recovery-guidance-document-2018-to-2020.pdf (Accessed 30 January 2025).

Health Service Executive (2024) *A National framework for Recovery in Mental Health 2024–2028* (Internet) Available at: www.hse.ie/eng/services/list/4/mental-health-servi ces/mental-health-engagement-and-recovery/resources-information-and-publications/a-national-framework-for-recovery-in-mental-health.pdf (Accessed 30 January 2025).

Maynooth University (2024) *MU Expert Recommends Whole-Family Approach to Mental Health Care* (Internet). Available at: www.maynoothuniversity.ie/all-institute/news/mu-expert-recommends-whole-family-approach-mental-health-care (Accessed 30 January 2025).

NHS Health Education England (2020) *The Competence framework for Mental Health Peer Support Workers* (Internet). Available at: www.hee.nhs.uk/sites/default/files/docume nts/The%20Competence%20Framework%20for%20MH%20PSWs%20-%20Part%20 1%20-%20Supporting%20document_0.pdf (Accessed 30 January 2025).

Norton, M.J. & Cullen, O.J. (2024) Recovery in mental health, addiction and dual diagnosis. In *Different Diagnoses, Similar Experiences: Narratives of Mental Health, Addiction Recovery and Dual Diagnosis* (Norton, M.J. & Cullen, O.J. eds.). Emerald Publishing Limited, Leeds, pp. 35–41.

Norton, M.J. & Cuskelly, K. (2021) Family recovery interventions with families of mental health service users: A systematic review of the literature. *International Journal of Environmental Research and Public Health* 18, 7858. https://doi.org/10.3390/ijerph.18157858

Office of Mental Health Engagement and Recovery, Mental Health Ireland and REFOCUS (2018) *A Family Recovery Resources Guide: Coproduced Content for Services and Organisations Supporting Families Living with Mental Health Challenges* (Internet). Available at: www.hse.ie/eng/services/list/4/mental-health-services/mental-health-eng agement-and-recovery/family-carer-and-supporter-guide/family-recovery-resource-guide-pdf.pdf (Accessed 30 January 2025).

Orygen (n.d.) *Fact Sheet: Family Peer Support and Youth Mental Health* (Internet). Available at: www.orygen.org.au/Training/Resources/Peer-work/Fact-sheets/Family-peer-support-youth-mental-health/orygen_family_peer_work_fact_sheet.aspx?ext= (Accessed 30 January 2025).

Our Community (2023). *Our Community* (Internet). Available at: www.ourcommunity.com. au/files/OCP/Section%20Eight.pdf (Accessed 31 August 2024).

Pachowicz, M. & Goffe, A. (2024) *Family Peer Support Work: A Review of Irish and International Literature* (Internet). Available at: www.tasc.ie/assets/files/pdf/family_peer _support_work_november_2024.pdf (Accessed 30 January 2025).

Reynolds, D. (2018) *Experiences of Receiving a Peer Support Intervention for Family Members of Individuals with Mental Illness* (Clinical Psychology Doctoral Dissertation), University of Limerick, Limerick, Ireland.

The Housing Agency (2024) *Peer Support Models: Examining Models both Nationally and Internationally* (Internet). Available at: www.housingagency.ie/sites/default/files/ 2024-12/The%20Housing%20Agency%20-%20Action%202.2.3%20a%20Peer%20 Support%20Models_0.pdf (Accessed 30 January 2025).

Appendix: Family Peer Support Worker Sample Job Description

Job Title, Grade Code	**Family Peer Support Worker** *(Grade code:)*
Campaign Reference	
Closing Date	
Proposed Interview Date (s)	
Taking Up Appointment	
Location of Post	
Informal Enquiries	**Name of the Manager:** **Email:** **Phone:**
Details of Service	
Reporting Relationship	
Key Working Relationships	
Purpose of the Post	
Principal Duties and Responsibilities	*Under the direction of the nominated line manager the Family Peer will:* • Build supportive and respectful relationships with families. • Encourage families to focus on their own wellness. • Act as a role model to family members to inspire hope and share experiences as a family member in recovery. • Assist family members to identify their needs strengths, personal interests, and goals. • Facilitate family members to learn new ways of communicating and problem-solving. • Assume a 'coaching' role supporting Family members in developing personal recovery plans. • Provide opportunities for Family members to direct their own recovery based on the recovery principles of 'hope', 'choice' and opportunity. • Provide relevant and reliable information on a wide range of mental health-related issues relevant to the family member's needs. • Signpost families to appropriate local support and information services in the community. • Assist Family members to understand their rights and choices within the service, including support with the care planning process where required, and the supports available to access these.

Job Title, Grade Code	Family Peer Support Worker *(Grade code:)*
	• Where the Relative has consented – support the family member in contributing to the care and treatment plan. • Liaise and co-operate with colleagues and wider Community Healthcare. • Manage a caseload in consultation with their line manager. • Report any incidents, complaints or concerns to their line manager/Supervisor. • To find ways to work as independently as possible in line in line with organisational policy. • Participate in regular supervision sessions and work with Supervisor to ensure that they are working effectively, and that their client's progress is relevant to their individual needs. • Attend Group Supervision and other meetings with mental health staff. • Promote equality of opportunity and good relations as outlined in the HSE Equality Policy. • Be aware of the Human Rights legislation in relation to the requirements of this post.
Eligibility Criteria Qualifications and/or Experience	**Candidates must have by the closing date for receipt of applications for this post:** **1. Requirements for the post, experience etc.** (a) Personal experience of mental health difficulties in one's family or close relationship including insight into the family recovery process **AND** (b) Experience of working (paid or voluntary) with individuals or families with mental health needs **AND/OR** **(c)** Hold a recognised training in Peer support or equivalent. **2. Health** A candidate for and any person holding the office must be fully competent and capable of undertaking the duties attached to the office and be in a state of health such as would indicate a reasonable prospect of ability to render regular and efficient service. **3. Character** Each candidate for and any person holding the office must uphold the values of recovery and the core values of the organisation.

(Continued)

Job Title, Grade Code	**Family Peer Support Worker** *(Grade code:)*
Post Specific Requirements	• Demonstrate depth and breadth of experience working with individuals/families with mental health needs as relevant to the role. • Demonstrate experience in the implementation of self-care frameworks and approaches in the context of mental health recovery, as relevant to the role.
Other Requirements Specific to the Post	• Access to transport is a necessary requirement to carry out the duties and responsibilities of this post as this is a role that requires the post holder to work from a variety of locations. • Ability to work in a flexible way, which may include evenings, weekends, bank and public holidays. • Post holders must be willing to complete specified training, and to continually develop the Family Peer Support Worker role.
Skills, Competencies and/or Knowledge	**Candidates must:** **Knowledge relevant to the role** • Demonstrate knowledge of the basic structure of the Community Mental Health Team. • Demonstrate knowledge of the organisation's Mental Health Services and organisational reform and change. • Demonstrate knowledge of the XXX mental health policy and the organisation's recovery framework and similar documentation. • Demonstrate knowledge of family recovery as a process and how to use their own recovery narrative to support others. • Demonstrate knowledge and understanding of the importance of self-care and associated techniques, from a recovery perspective. • Demonstrate knowledge and experience in co-facilitating a variety of group activities that support and strengthen Family recovery. • Demonstrate knowledge of current best practices in mental health recovery and social inclusion. Demonstrate a basic working knowledge of Information Technology, i.e., Microsoft Office (Word/PowerPoint) Google Docs, Social media platforms **Planning and Organising Skills** • Demonstrate organisational and time management skills to meet objectives within agreed timeframes and achieve quality results

Job Title, Grade Code	Family Peer Support Worker *(Grade code:)*
	• Demonstrate the ability to work to tight deadlines and operate effectively with multiple competing priorities. **Evaluating Information and Decision-Making** • Demonstrate the ability to assess complex information from a variety of sources and make effective decisions. • Demonstrate effective problem-solving and decision-making skills. **Leadership and Teamwork** • Demonstrate teamwork skills including the ability to work with a broad range of professionals and agencies. • Demonstrate a capacity to operate successfully in a challenging operational environment while adhering to quality standards. • Demonstrate motivation and an innovative approach to the job within a changing working environment. • Demonstrate the ability to co-facilitate groups. • Demonstrate the ability to be flexible and adapt to change. • Demonstrate ability to work as a lone worker, in a range of settings and as appropriate. **Commitment to Providing a Quality Service** • Demonstrate a person-centred focus in the delivery of services. • Demonstrate a core belief in and passion for the sustainable delivery of high-quality user-focused and family-friendly services. • Demonstrate a commitment to recovery-focused community development principles and practices. • Demonstrate commitment to continuing learning and development. **Communication and Interpersonal Skills** • Demonstrate effective interpersonal skills. • Demonstrate effective written and verbal communication skills; including the ability to present information in a clear and concise manner. • Demonstrate ability to form peer relationships with service users and family members. • Demonstrate the ability to interact in a professional manner with other Mental Health staff and other key stakeholders.

(Continued)

Job Title, Grade Code	Family Peer Support Worker *(Grade code:)*
Campaign-Specific Selection Process Ranking/Shortlisting/ Interview	
Code of Practice	
This Job Specification is a guide to the general range of duties assigned to the post holder. It is intended to be neither definitive nor restrictive and is subject to periodic review with the employee concerned.	

Chapter 12

Peer Support Work Specialisms

12.1 Introduction

This chapter marks the second of three examining the practice of peer support work within mental health service provision. Peer support work is an ever-growing practice that has been introduced within different contexts like that of family peer work, forensic services as well as other, more synchronous services only available online (Shalaby and Agyapong, 2020; Fortuna et al., 2022; Mikolajczak-Degrauwe et al., 2023). In this chapter, we explore the various contexts in which peer support work is practised in mental health. We begin this by exploring peer support work in child and adolescent mental health services (CAMHS). This is followed by peer support within forensic services as presented in Section 12.3. Section 12.4 explores the role when working with unique communities. Section 12.5 concludes the chapter by providing a synopsis of what we have learned.

12.2 Child and Adolescent Mental Health (CAMHS)

CAMHS are specialist mental health services specifically designed to meet the needs of young people up to the age of 18 years who experience moderate-to-severe mental health challenges (Mental Health Commission, 2023). However, in recent years, such services have been confronted with an ever-increasing number of young people experiencing severe and enduring mental health challenges, although pharmacological and other psychotherapeutic interventions alone are insufficient in responding to this growing demand (European Society for Child and Adolescent Psychiatry, 2023). This shortage in resources can lead to poor service management, as is the case with Irish CAMHS services currently, which have been described as fragmented and overstretched with poor resources and staffing levels as common issues (Rooney et al., 2021; Mental Health Reform, 2023).

Within the wider mental health discourse, peer support work has also been evident in different ways even for young people experiencing mental health difficulties (Coleman et al., 2017). In this chapter, we focus on formalised Youth Peer Support Workers, who, like their adult peer colleagues, have experienced mental distress during childhood and/or adolescence but now utilise those experiences

DOI: 10.4324/9781032717050-17

to help other young people in similar circumstances and earlier phases of their recovery (de Beer et al., 2024a). Despite working with young people, their role is very similar to that of adult Peer Support Workers. However, interestingly, their ability to create an informal space filled with mutuality and reciprocity is not necessarily similar to that of the methodology that adult peers utilise to create informality. Here, Youth Peer Support Workers utilise their youthfulness as key to the creation of a connection needed for peer support to work with this cohort (de Beer et al., 2024b). In creating informality, Youth Peer Support Workers ignite hope whilst also manifesting destigmatisation and acting as a catalyst to create culturally and developmentally appropriate services (de Beer et al., 2023). Although services note some crossover of roles between disciplines, youth peer support work is unique in the sense that it emphasises the need for the participation of children and young people in not only their own care but also in reshaping traditional mental health service provision (Archard et al., 2023). However, it is important to note that evidence regarding Youth Peer Support Workers' effectiveness to those they serve is yet limited (Norton et al., 2023).

12.3 Forensic Mental Health Services

Forensic mental health is a specialised branch of mental health services which is dedicated to assessing and treating those individuals who are mentally unwell, but also those who, in some way, are involved in the criminal justice system – either in a prison or in a secure, approved forensic psychiatric facility (Finnerty and Gilheaney, n.d.). It is a service that primarily should be delivered on a regional basis dependent on the distribution of the prison population across regions (Mental Health Commission, 2006). Indeed, forensic mental health services have, in recent years, grown to be more structured and complex in their processes and pathways to care (Kennedy, 2022). Despite this, in the most recent model of care for forensic mental health services in Ireland, the importance of developing peer support work within such services is noted as paramount, particularly from the patient's perspective (Health Service Executive, 2019).

Forensic Peer Support Workers are individuals who experience both mental health challenges and incarceration by utilising these experiences to instil hope and act as role models for those in an earlier phase of recovery (Davidson and Rowe, 2008). They are useful, particularly, after when the acute phase of mental health challenges has passed and the service user is actively working towards re-integrating back into the community after a period of incarceration (Norton et al., 2023). They support service users in this activity by promoting self-advocacy, inspiring hope and connecting service users with resources that they can use to educate themselves not just about their own mental health but also about the criminal justice system (Pennsylvania Mental Health Consumers' Association, 2025). Despite these positive benefits to the provision of care for service users, the same issues mentioned before – such as a lack of role clarity – remain problematic for the integration of the role into more restricted, acute, coercive environments (Adams and Lincoln, 2021; Nash et al., 2022). Additionally, structural issues, such as the over-restriction of service user activity while maintaining a safe environment, are another barrier to effective peer support work in these settings (Walde and Vollm, 2023; Hardy et al., 2024). However, forensic peer support work is important in this setting as it provides a valuable outlet for service users as contact with friends and family members is restricted and, therefore, limited (Walde et al., 2023). As such, more research is required for future scholars to understand its inner workings within the forensic mental health environment.

12.4 Unique Communities

Indeed, young people and forensic services are not the only services to be supported by the presence of Peer Support Workers. Wright and Mahon (2024) speak of peer support work for people with addiction challenges. Peer support services for addictions are not new (Tracy and Wallace, 2016) as there are a number of peer groups well established in this area to support individuals with addiction. Such groups include Alcoholics Anonymous,[1] Narcotics Anonymous[2] and SMART Recovery[3]. In Irish services, Better Together[4] was established to facilitate peer support for individuals in addiction and is growing in popularity across the Republic of Ireland today.

Apart from addiction services, peer support has also been established for people experiencing homelessness (O'Donnell and Cusack, 2024). The reason behind this approach is that those who experience homelessness are often the individuals with the most complex social and health issues (Miler et al., 2020). As a result, in 2024, The Housing Agency published a toolkit to support homelessness services in training, recruiting and sustaining peer support roles within this setting (The Housing Agency, 2024). However, before this, Hail[5] – a housing agency situated in Dublin, Ireland – commenced a peer support project in 2016 where they trained peers to the same standard as those peers in the health service and then employed them to run the project with huge success (Hail, 2025).

Peer support work has also been implemented within ethnic minority communities (Usideme, 2024), which is inclusive of the travelling community (Harty, 2024). A peer service dedicated specifically to ethnic minorities and travellers is not yet fully developed. However, within Irish mental health services, 1 of the 30 Peer Support Workers employed by the statutory services is a traveller who now works specifically with the travelling community (Dublin City University, 2023; Health Service Executive, 2023). However, in the near future, further development is needed to interact with these communities, as well as with ethnic minorities and traveller communities, as the key to understanding and supporting them with their mental health is to understand their culture, which grounds their identity (Behavioral Health Workforce Development, 2023). Moreover, it is necessary to recruit more peers from these communities so that these unique members of our society can be better served.

12.5 Concluding Remarks

In summary, this chapter explored specialist areas of practice within peer support work, some of which are only still developing in an Irish context. We began the chapter by exploring Youth Peer Support Workers and how they engage with children and adolescents up to 18 years. Next, we examined Forensic Peer Support Workers who primarily work with individuals who experienced mental health challenges and are currently incarcerated either within the prison system or in a secure, approved psychiatric facility. Here, we found that evidence of effectiveness was sparse. Lastly, we examined peer support work within a variety of unique communities, including those with addiction, homelessness, as well as those from ethnic minority and traveller communities. We also explored specialist peer support work (including the last chapter on family peer support work). In the following chapter, 'Current Peer Support Practices', we will explore current practices in peer work that have been captured from the case studies in the earlier chapters.

Notes

1   www.alcoholicsanonymous.ie/
2   www.na-ireland.org/
3   https://smartrecovery.ie/
4   https://better-together.ie/
5   https://hail.ie/

References

Adams, W.E. & Lincoln, A.K. (2021) Barriers to and facilitators of implementing peer support services for criminal justice-involved individuals. *Psychiatric Services* 72(6), 626–632. https://doi.org/10.1176/appi.ps.201900627

Archard, P.J., O'Reilly, M., Spilsbury, T., Ali, A., Kulik, L. & Solanki, P. (2023) Informality, advocacy and the sharing of lived experience in peer support work. *Irish Journal of Psychological Medicine.* https://doi.org/10.1017/ipm.2023.8

Behavioral Health Workforce Development (2023) *Supporting Equity through Peer Support* (Internet). Available at: www.workforce.buildingcalhhs.com/resource/supporting-equity-through-peer-support/ (Accessed 05 February 2025).

Coleman, N., Sykes, W. & Groom, C. (2017) *Peer Support and Children and Young People's Mental Health: Research Review* (Internet). Available at: https://assets.publishing.serv ice.gov.uk/media/5a820b3d40f0b62305b922c5/Children_and_young_people_s_men tal_health_peer_support.pdf (Accessed 04 February 2025).

Davidson, L. & Rowe, M. (2008) *Peer Support within Criminal Justice Settings: The Role of Forensic Peer Specialists* (Internet). Available at: www.fredla.org/wp-content/uploads/2016/01/davidsonrowe_peersupport1.pdf (Accessed 05 February 2025).

de Beer, C.R.M., Nooteboom, L.A., van Domburgh, L., de Vreugd, M., Schoones, J.W. & Vermeiren, R.R.J.M. (2024a) A systematic review exploring youth peer support for young people with mental health problems. *European Child and Adolescent Psychiatry* 33, 2471–2484. https://doi.org/10.1007/s00787-022-02120-5

de Beer, C.R.M., Vermeiren, R.R.J.M., Nooteboom, L.A., Kuiper, C.H.Z., Groenendijk, J.C.M.L., de Vreugd, M. & van Domburgh, L. (2024b) A balancing act: Integrating the expertise of youth peer workers in child and adolescent mental health services. *European Child and Adolescent Psychiatry*. https://doi.org/10.1007/s00 787-024-02498-4

de Beer, C.R.M., van Domburgh, L., Vermeiren, R.R.J.M., de Vreugd, M. & Nooteboom, L.A. (2023) Improving collaboration between youth peer support workers and non-peer colleagues in child and adolescent mental health services. *Administration and Policy in Mental Health and Mental Health Services Research* 50, 824–833. https://doi.org/10.1007/s10488-023-01283-w

Dublin City University (2023) *Julie Duke* (Internet). Available at: https://www.dcu.ie/community-profiles/julie-duke (Accessed 05 February 2025).

European Society for Child and Adolescent Psychiatry (2023) *Involving Youth Peer Support Workers in Child and Adolescent Psychiatry* (Internet). Available at: www.escap.eu/division/policy-division/youth-peer-support-workers (Accessed 04 February 2025).

Finnerty, S & Gilheaney, P. (n.d.) *Access to Mental Health Services for People in the Criminal Justice System* (Internet). Available at: www.mhcirl.ie/sites/default/files/2021-11/Acc ess%20to%20mental%20health%20services%20for%20people%20in%20the%20crimi nal%20justice%20system%20FINAL.pdf (Accessed 05 February 2025).

Fortuna, K.L., Solomon, P. & Rivera, J. (2022) An update of peer support/peer provided services underlying processes, benefits and critical ingredients. *Psychiatry Quarterly* 93, 571–586. https://doi.org/10.1007/s11126-022-09971-w

Hail, (2025) *Peer Support Project* (Internet). Available at: https://hail.ie/support-services/peer-support-project/ (Accessed 05 February 2025).

Hardy, S.C., Alves-Costa, F. & Robinson, G. (2024) Peer support-led interventions in forensic settings: Listening to service users and peer support workers' perceptions and experiences. *Journal of Forensic Psychology Research and Practice* 24(5), 771–793. https://doi.org/10.1080/24732850.2023.2251446

Harty, M. (2024) Peer support work within the traveller community. In *Peer Support Work: Practice, Training and Implementation* (Mahon, D. eds.). Emerald Publishing Limited, Leeds, pp. 83–94.

Health Service Executive (2019) *National Forensic Mental Health Services: Model of Care*. Health Service Executive, Ireland.

Health Service Executive (2023) *Mental Health Engagement and Recovery Office Strategic Plan 2023-2026: Engaged in Recovery* (Internet). Available at: www.hse.ie/eng/services/list/4/mental-health-services/mental-health-engagement-and-recovery/mher-strategic-plan-engaged-in-recovery.pdf (Accessed 05 February 2025).

Kennedy, H.G. (2022) Models of care in forensic psychiatry. *BJPsych Advances* 28, 46–59. https://doi.org/10.1192/bja.2021.34

Mental Health Commission (2006) *Forensic Mental Health Services for Adults in Ireland* (Internet). Available at: www.lenus.ie/bitstream/handle/10147/43831/4368.pdf?seque nce–1&isAllowed=y (Accessed 05 February 2025).

Mental Health Commission (2023) *Independent Review of the Provision of Child and Adolescent Mental Health Services (CAMHS) in the State by the Inspector of Mental Health Services* (Internet). Available at: www.mhcirl.ie/sites/default/files/2023-07/Men tal%20Health%20Commission%20Independent%20Reviews%20of%20CAMHS%20s ervices%20in%20the%20State.pdf (Accessed 04 February 2025).

Mental Health Reform (2023) *Mental Health Commission's CAMHS Review Reveals Risks to Children's Safety* (Internet). Available at: https://mentalhealthreform.ie/news/mental -health-commissions-camhs-review-reveals-risks-to-childrens-safety/ (Accessed 04 February 2025).

Mikolajczak-Degrauwe, K., Slimmen, S.R., Gillissen, D., de Bil, P., Bosmans, V., Keemink, C., Meyvis, I. & Kuipers, Y.J. (2023) Strengths, weaknesses, opportunities and threats of peer support among disadvantaged groups: A rapid scoping review. *International Journal of Nursing Science* 10(4), 587–601. https://doi.org/10.1016/j.ijnss.2023.09.002

Miler, J.A., Carver, H., Foster, R. & Parkes, T. (2020) Provision of peer support at the intersection of homelessness and problem substance use services: A systematic 'state of the art' review. *BMC Public Health* 20, 641. https://doi.org/10.1186/s12889-020-8407-4

Nash, E., Taplin, S., Rust, L.J. & Percival, R. (2022) Staff experiences of working alongside peer support workers in forensic mental health community teams: A qualitative study. *Journal of Forensic Practice* 24(4), 354–363. https://doi.org/10.1108/JFP-05-2021-0030

Norton, M.J., Clabby, P., Coyle, B., Cruickshank, J., Davidson, G., Greer, K., Kilcommins, M., McCartan, C., McGuire, E., McGilloway, S., Mulholland, C., O'Connell-Gannon, M., Pepper, D., Shannon, C., Swords, C., Walsh, J. & Webb, P. (2023) *Peer Support Work: An International Scoping Review* (Internet). Available at: https://pureadmin.qub.ac.uk/ws/portalfiles/portal/543700214/Peer_Support_Work_Scoping_Review_Main_report.pdf (Accessed 04 February 2025).

O'Donnell, C. & Cusack, A. (2024) Homelessness and peer work. In *Peer Support Work: Practice, Training and Implementation* (Mahon, D. eds.). Emerald Publishing Limited, Leeds, pp. 43–57.

Pennsylvania Mental Health Consumers' Association (2025) *FPS Training* (Internet). Available at: https://pmhca.wildapricot.org/Peer-Support-Within-the-Criminal-Justice-System-Forensic-Peer-Support (Accessed 05 February 2025).

Rooney, L., Harrold, A., McNicholas, F., Gavin, B., Cullen, W. & Quigley, E. (2021) Child and adolescent mental health service: Extension for community health care options [CAMHS ECHO]. *Irish Medical Journal* 114(1), 241.

Shalaby, R.A.H. & Agyapong, V.I.O. (2020) Peer support in mental health: Literature review. *JMIR Mental Health* 7(6), e15572. https://doi.org/10.2196/15572

The Housing Agency (2024) *Peer Support Specialist Toolkit: Integration and Delivery of Peer Support Specialist Services* (Internet). Available at: www.housingagency.ie/sites/default/files/2024-09/The%20Housing%20Agency%20103982_Peer%20Support%20Specialist%20Toolkit_FINAL.pdf (Accessed 05 February 2025).

Tracy, K. & Wallace, S.P. (2016) Benefits of peer support groups in the treatment of addiction. *Substance Abuse and Rehabilitation* 143–154. https://doi.org/10.2147/SAR.S81535

Usideme, O.I. (2024) Peer work in ethnic minorities communities. In *Peer Support Work: Practice, Training and Implementation* (Mahon, D. eds.). Emerald Publishing Limited, Leeds, pp. 73–82.

Walde, P., Hadala, J., Peipe, V. & Vollm, B.A. (2023) Implementation of a peer support worker in a forensic psychiatric hospital in Germany – Views of patients. *Frontiers in Psychiatry* 14, 1061106. https://doi.org/10.3389/fpsyt.2023.1061106

Walde, P. & Vollm, B. (2023) What does a peer support worker do in a forensic mental health clinic for addicted offenders. *European Psychiatry* 66(Suppl 1), S882. https://doi.org/10.1192/j.eurpsy.2023.1868

Wright, M. & Mahon, D. (2024) Addiction and peer support work. In *Peer Support Work: Practice, Training and Implementation* (Mahon, D. eds.). Emerald Publishing Limited, Leeds, pp. 25–34.

Chapter 13

Current Peer Support Practices

13.1 Introduction

In the previous two chapters, we explored peer support specialisms and their potential to make a difference in their various fields. Although the progression of peer support roles from simply being involved in general adult mental health services to such specialisms is an important milestone in terms of building a profession, one must not lose focus in the development of a discipline/profession. Instead, the peer should focus on the simplicity of the practice and the process of perfecting it as it allows for it to be most effective. However, the creation of specialisms is important in bringing this simplicity to other, less marginalised communities along the health trajectory. But it is important to re-iterate that we do not overlook what makes peer support unique in the search for professionalisation. This chapter winds up the discussion on the practice of peer support work. For this, we will examine current peer support practices through an in-depth exploration of the nine case studies that supported the creation of this book. This process begins in Section 13.2 where the process of creating this in-depth discussion will be discussed, followed by the discussion on current practice. It also explores the methodology behind Braun and Clarke's (2006, 2019, 2022, 2024) reflexive thematic analysis. Section 13.3 concludes the chapter.

13.2 Braun and Clarke's Reflexive Thematic Analysis

As a methodological approach, the process of reflexive thematic analysis was developed from the work of Virginia Braun and Victoria Clarke over the past 20 years (Norton and Cullen, 2024). The process is useful for qualitative synthesis and consists of six key steps (Norton, 2023, 2024), which are described in detail in Table 13.1.

From utilising this methodological tool on the nine case studies, four themes were constructed – '*places of employment*', '*peer support roles*', '*benefits of peer support work*' and '*challenges to authentic peer support work*'. Please note that more themes were created from utilising this approach, but in keeping with the focus of this chapter, I will only discuss the themes and sub-themes related to

DOI: 10.4324/9781032717050-18

Table 13.1 Six Key Steps to Braun and Clarke's Reflexive Thematic Analysis

Phase Number	Phase Description	Explanation of Phase
1.	**Familiarisation with the data**	Involves a deep, intimate understanding of the data set. The analyst engages with the information in a way that allows for both immersion and distance from the data to occur. Immersion allows for an intimate understanding of the data. Distance from the data allows for critical engagement with the data.
2.	**Coding the data**	The analyst works through each data item, reads it and notes what is relevant under generic codes.
3.	**Generating initial themes**	Incorporates a reflective process where codes are generated and revisited many times until clusters form and initial lists of themes are constructed from the data set.
4.	**Reviewing and developing themes**	This phase checks on the work already conducted through a re-engagement with both coded data and the entire data set. The purpose is to review the initial clusters and reflect to identify if better patterns should be developed.
5.	**Refining, defining and naming themes**	Themes are further developed through an analytical write-up of these themes derived from the data set. This allows the analyst to explore the themes and identify the way in which they should present the constructed themes.
6.	**Producing the report**	One continues to develop the themes from the data, even as the report is being written up. As such, this final stage involves deep refining analytical work that allows the analyst to shape the work and ensure that the analysis flows well.

Source: Six key steps originated from Braun and Clarke (2022).

Table 13.2 Constructed Themes and Associated Sub-Themes

Themes	Sub-Themes
Places of employment	
Peer support roles	Lived experience as knowledge
	Emotional support
	Reflection
Benefits of peer support work	Dual role
	Approachability
Challenges to authentic peer support work	Working under a biomedical system
	Constraint towards honesty and authenticity
	Lack of opportunities for career progression

current peer support practice. These themes and their associated sub-themes are presented in the following sections (Table 13.2).

13.2.1 Places of Employment

Four peers from the nine case studies work for a statutory mental health service. Peers have been placed in acute wards (x2), within an NHS (National Health Service)-funded recovery college (x1) and within the specialist area of child and adolescent mental health services (CAMHS) (x1). The remaining peers are placed within the non-governmental, voluntary sector. Placements included a peer-led service, a peer support group, a recovery college not funded by statutory services and a mental health charity.

13.2.2 Peer Support Roles

Within the theme of peer support roles come three sub-themes: '*lived experience as knowledge*', '*emotional support*' and '*reflection*'. These are the most prominent roles of the Peer Support Worker currently being used today within service provision. Firstly, when the Peer Support Worker first meets the individual, there is often '*... a barrier ... to break through so [that the service user] would see [the peer] as different from other staff*'. Often '*... the fastest and most effective way to do that is to share [their] own [lived] experience ...*'. This allows peers, unlike their non-peer counterparts, to become suitably '*... equipped to notice cultural or interpersonal issues that others might miss*' due to their unique knowledge set. However, '*... sharing [ones] lived experiences needs to be done with caution*' as if doing it incorrectly '*... can compromise rapport building and connection...*'. In this way '*... there are [certain] boundaries that [one should] not cross...*'. Rachael gives an example about sharing her experiences of living with anorexia nervosa, stating that she would

> *never share numbers – weight, calories, admission number, body mass index (BMI)… graphic depictions such as photos or explicit stories. [She also would not]… delve into the details of [her] most distressing traumas nor will [she] share 'before and after' comparisons.*

However, despite the potential of destroying the peer relationship, such experiences are ultimately shared to '…*establish more informal relationship[s] grounded on some commonality'*. However, '… *there's no distinct model behind it…*". Despite this,

> *there are countless … opportunities available for individuals to support each other and for peers to intervene when self-disclosure is needed to increase self-empowerment of individuals. Such opportunities [include]: guided group discussions …[and] casual conversations … [over] tea and coffee.*

Regardless of how it is shared, Lydia documents the results of such interaction for all parties involved:

> *When someone shares their experiences, no matter how unusual or difficult they may seem, our first response is to validate. This does not mean we agree with every perspective or experience, but it does mean we acknowledge that every person's feelings are real and worthy of recognition… Recognition, then is about seeing the person behind the struggles, acknowledging their contributions and celebrating their strengths even in moments of vulnerability.*

This quotation from Lydia's case study demonstrates that when lived experience is shared '… *in a positive way, [it] create[s] a ripple effect that sets mental health recovery in motion'*. The use of lived experience in this way '… *adds another layer to healing – one that many don't get to encounter – to use pain for something positive*". For Rachael, this lived experience knowledge is something that not everyone can possess unlike learned knowledge. Here Rachael suggests that lived experience is not something that can be achieved via class, activity or a textbook. It is something more personal, more meaningful than what learnt knowledge can ever possess:

> *Whilst jumping through the hoops of courses and certification is still often a necessity in the peer space, it is not the primary qualification. Rather it is lived experience – a personal level of understanding far beyond what can be laid out by a set curriculum. Textbooks and articles and academic titles only account for so much.*

When a Peer Support Worker is not sharing their lived experiences, they also carry out a number of roles under the banner of emotional support. Such tasks include '... *attending community meetings ... providing messages to consumers of activities for participation ... co-facilitate consumer advisory groups...[and] discussing what issues that were most important to them ...*'. Such emotional support also included '... *provid[ing] various coping mechanisms that ...*' worked for peers in the past. Finally, '... *Peer Support Worker[s]... often question [where they are at in their] own personal recovery and how ...to continue to look after [themselves], whilst helping others on their journey too*'. This process is considered an act of reflection within the peer role. It is an important characteristic for peers to adapt because it '...*can sometimes [allow the peer to] feel more connected to client's experiences ...*' which is an important aspect of '... *validat[ing] their experiences]*'.

13.2.3 Benefits of Peer Support Work

In terms of benefits of peer support work, the case studies have noted two such benefits: '*dual role*' and '*approachability*'. As noted in earlier discussions, Peer Support Workers sit in a tenuous space that occupies both professionalisation and friendship. Within the case studies collected, this space is clearly evident. This dual role is beneficial for the peer as they '... *can see things from both perspectives*'. The side of the '... *overworked tired professional ...*' and the '... *experience of living this for myself...*'. In this way, the peer relationship extends '... *beyond professional interactions*' into something more intimate. Although both sides of the tenuous relationship may '... *sometimes complement each other... [but] fulfilling both roles can be multi-faceted and complex, especially when flipping from various perspectives all in one day*'. Nina explains this complexity of this tenuous space in the following quotation:

> I was so scared staff would see me as a patient but at the same time scared that the residents would see me as a normal member of staff.

Another benefit of peer support work is the approachability of the Peer Support Worker. For Lydia, being approachable meant

> being available for others, without rushing to a solution or offering unasked-for advice ... This requires ... constantly check[ing] in with our biases and assumptions ... By ensuring that approachability is central to our ethos ... a [relationship is created] where no one feels isolated in their struggles, and everyone feels respected and heard.

13.2.4 Challenges to Authentic Peer Support Work

The final theme constructed from these case studies is the challenges to authentic peer support work. The case studies identified three main sub-themes: '*working under a biomedical system*', '*constraint towards honesty and authenticity*' and finally '*lack of opportunity for career progression*'. These sub-themes are presented in the following sections.

The first sub-theme is '*working under a biomedical system*'. Within the case studies, two major issues arose from working under a biomedical system. The first involved the ethos of a biomedical system itself. This consists of '*working with people who immediately reel off a list of diagnosis…*'. This creates a challenge to the peer as they '*… understand the power of vulnerability*' that comes from the use of such an approach. Another case study contributor explains how this also challenges them:

> *because I feel like I need to unpick everything that has happened to them to understand them as a human and not as a set of symptoms. That of course creates some internal conflict as most people go to the NHS to get a diagnosis and usually medicine to manage their symptoms and it is not my job to unpick their diagnosis.*

Another difficulty comes from the expectation of the peer '*… to have it all together…*' and to '*… present as 'recovered' rather than as someone who understands what care may look like and offer a non-oppressive opinion…*'; this has led this contributor to feel like peer work is being presented tokenistically to try to prove the point that the services actually work and not to do what the role was created for which is '*… to advocate and try to change the system that may have caused them harm*' in the first place.

The biomedical system can also restrain the peer from actually expressing themselves fully. One contributor noted, '*when [they] did peer work unofficially, [they] had less constraints and could be more honest about what [they] thought about the system [they] now work in*'. However, now as they are professionals, it '*… comes with rules and expectations of how a professional communicates and behaves*''. Another contributor noted that it is possible to acknowledge this but this can threaten career progression. This is even though '*… progression [whilst] keeping [one's] lived experience [is] limited*'. Additionally, due to a lack of understanding regarding the informality of peer work within traditional discourse, bullying from other staff – peer or non-peer – can ensue as noted in Matthew's case study:

> *The outgoing carer consultant clashed with my new ideas and more progressive and inclusive approach to work more collaboratively with the consumer consultant team … Because of the personal clash … she went around telling other carers she worked with, my future peers I was supposed to support didn't like me, effectively sabotaging the role I was taking over … she was bullying me behind my back. This escalated to human resources, and I had a major complex trauma response.*

13.3 Concluding Remarks

In summary, this chapter – the last to discuss the practice of peer support work – documents the results of a process of reflexive thematic analysis on the nine case studies collected for this book, from which four themes and eight sub-themes were constructed. Each of these examined aspects of current peer support practice from across the world. Of interest is the use of lived experience and the pure lack of a universal mechanism for its use. Another interesting finding is how the traditional system can constrain natural peer support activity, raising the question of whether Peer Support Workers should work in such restricted environments. The next – final – chapter will provide a synopsis of the learnings from creating and reading this text as well as some helpful resources for establishing and growing peer support within your mental health service.

References

Braun, V. & Clarke, V. (2006) Using thematic analysis in psychology. *Qualitative Research in Psychology* 3(2), 77–101.

Braun, V. & Clarke, V. (2019) Reflecting on reflexive thematic analysis. *Qualitative Research in Sport, Exercise and Health* 11(4), 589–597. https://doi.org/10.1080/21596 76X.2019.1628806

Braun, V. & Clarke, V. (2022) *Thematic Analysis: A Practical Guide.* SAGE Publications Limited, London.

Braun, V. & Clarke, V. (2024) Supporting best practice in reflexive thematic analysis reporting in palliative medicine: A review of published research and introduction to the reflexive thematic analysis reporting guidelines (RTARG). *Palliative Medicine* 38(6), 608–616. https://doi.org/10.1177/02692163241234800

Norton, M.J. (2023) *A National Framework for Mental Health Engagement and Recovery: A Co-Designed Measurement Tool.* Masters Dissertation, Royal College of Surgeons in Ireland, Dublin, Ireland.

Norton, M.J. (2024) *Family Recovery in Child and Adolescent Mental Health: A Systematic Review.* Masters Dissertation, Dublin City University, Dublin, Ireland.

Norton, M.J. & Cullen, O.J. (2024) Fusing experiences, reflexive thematic analysis. In *Different Diagnoses, Similar Experiences: Narratives of Mental Health, Addiction Recovery and Dual Diagnosis* (Norton, M.J & Cullen, O.J. eds.). Emerald Publishing Limited, Leeds, pp. 177–206.

Part 6

Concluding Remarks

Chapter 14

Conclusion

14.1 Introduction

Being the final chapter of this text, its purpose is to provide a synopsis of each chapter of this text. Additionally, the chapter will also provide some helpful resources to support service managers who wish to implement peer support work to do so. Such resources include YouTube videos produced by the Office of Mental Health Engagement and Recovery and Genio into the role. It also contains useful guides, literature reviews and toolkits that can support any service thinking of implementing peer support to do so. Section 14.2 provides a synopsis of each chapter of this text.

14.2 Synopsis of Each Chapter of This Text

The following is a brief summary of each chapter of this text.

1. **Chapter 1: Context: Setting the Scene** – It starts to set the scene by exploring the current state of peer support globally whilst also examining the evidence base for the same within mental health service provision. The chapter also discusses the purpose of this text, laying in motion the chapters to follow.
2. **Chapter 2: Historical Underpinnings of Mental Health Service Provision Inclusive of the History of the Peer Support Movement** – This chapter explores the history of both the mental health services and the peer support work movement within mental health discourse. The chapter also examines three models of understanding mental distress: biomedical, stress vulnerability and, finally, mental distress as a result of trauma.
3. **Chapter 3: Definitions of Peer Support Work** – This chapter explores various components of a definition of peer support work in mental health discourse to construct a new definition that can be used to more adequately define peer support work in mental health.
4. **Chapter 4: Principles and Roles of Peer Support Work** – This chapter explores the various principles, values, competencies and roles of Peer Support Workers identified in the literature thus far.

DOI: 10.4324/9781032717050-20

5. **Chapter 5: Advantages of and Challenges to Peer Support Work** – This chapter explores the various benefits and challenges to peer support work within mental health discourse from a micro to a macro level.

6. **Chapter 6: Experiential Knowledge/Lived Experience** – This chapter provides a detailed exploration into the knowledge set used by Peer Support Workers to support individual and organisational recovery outcomes.

7. **Chapter 7: Models of Peer Support Work** – This chapter explores two models of peer support work: '*The Stepping Model*' developed by the author and colleagues, and '*The Stepped Model of Peer Provider Practice*' created by Zeng and Chung (2019).

8. **Chapter 8: Ethical Dilemmas in Peer Support Work** – This chapter examines the various ethical issues/dilemmas relating to peer support work. Examples include the maintenance of a dual role, ethical informality and working in an environment where one was formally a patient.

9. **Chapter 9: Peer Support Work in Traditional Mental Health Discourse** – Chapter 9 examines the placement of Peer Support Workers in traditional mental health services and attempts to showcase the arguments for and against Peer Support Worker placements in such environments.

10. **Chapter 10: Policy Developments in Support of Peer Support Work** – This chapter explores the policy developments in several jurisdictions that have led to the introduction of Peer Support Workers in these areas. Jurisdictions include Ireland, the UK, the USA, Australia and China. The areas were chosen as a result of the proliferation of philosophical and theoretical debate into this specialist area of mental health service provision within these jurisdictions.

11. **Chapter 11: Family Peer Support Work** –This chapter explores the specialist role of family peer support work in mental health service provision. It also includes discussions on family recovery, defining family peer support work as well as discussing the unique referral process for Family Peer Support Workers given that they sit externally to the multi-disciplinary team. Finally, the chapter concludes with a list of recommendations and resources to advance family peer support work in mental health discourse.

12. **Chapter 12: Peer Support Work Specialisms** – This chapter explores the other specialisations of peer support work within child and adolescent mental health services, to forensic mental health and finally to that of unique communities within our society, including the traveller community.

13. **Chapter 13: Current Peer Support Practices** – This chapter utilises Braun and Clarke's reflexive thematic analysis to analyse the nine case studies included in this text to present a picture of current mental health service provision.

14.3 List of Helpful Resources

- Peer Support Workers HSE video – Office of Mental Health Engagement and Recovery: www.youtube.com/watch?v=YGlVrXJYM5c

- Family Peer Support Workers HSE video – Office of Mental Health Engagement and Recovery: www.youtube.com/watch?v=4sIlfHDiqcw
- Induction of Peer Support within the Health Service Executive – Office of Mental Health Engagement and Recovery/Genio: www.youtube.com/watch?v=PYUN4x2KhoE
- Toolkit to Support Peer Support Workers Working in the Health Service Executive – Office of Mental Health Engagement and Recovery:://www.hse.ie/eng/services/list/4/mental-health-services/mentalhealthengagement/peer-support-workers-toolkit.pdf
- Peer Support Worker: A Guidance Paper – Advancing Recovery in Ireland: www.lenus.ie/bitstream/handle/10147/576059/PeerSupportWorkersAGuidancePaper.pdf?sequence=6
- Family Peer Support Worker Website – Family Peer Support Network: https://familypeersupport.ie/
- Recovery Principles and Practice Training – Office of Mental Health Engagement and Recovery – Contact the Office at mhengage@hse.ie
- Intentional Peer Support – Sherry Mead: https://intentionalpeersupport.org/

Link to Eventbrite for Intentional Peer Support training: www.eventbrite.com/o/intentional-peer-support-20154714284

- Mahon, D. (2024) *Peer Support Work: Practice, Training and Implementation.* Emerald Publishing Limited, Leeds.
- Watson, E. & Meddings, S. (2019) *Peer Support in Mental Health.* Springer Red Globe Press, London.
- Implementing Recovery through Organisational Change [ImROC] –www.imroc.org/
- Norton, M.J., Clabby, P., Coyle, B., Cruickshank, J., Davidson, G., Greer, K., Kilcommins, M., McCartan, C., McGuire, E., McGilloway, S., Mulholland, C., O'Connell-Gannon, M., Pepper, D., Shannon, C., Swords, C., Walsh, J. & Webb, P. (2023) *Peer Support Work: An International Scoping Review* (Internet). Available at: https://pureadmin.qub.ac.uk/ws/portalfiles/portal/543700214/Peer_Support_Work_Scoping_Review_Main_report.pdf (Accessed 06 February 2025).
- Pachowicz, M. & Goffe, A. (2024) *Family Peer Support Work: A Review of Irish and International Literature* (Internet). Available at: www.tasc.ie/assets/files/pdf/family_peer_support_work_november_2024.pdf (Accessed 06 February 2025).

Please note that this list of helpful resources is non-exhaustive and centres primarily within an Irish/UK context. Please also be aware that peer support work resources may describe peer support differently in different jurisdictions, so please keep your own context in mind when reviewing the above resources.

Reference

Zeng, G. & Chung, D. (2019) The Stepped of Peer Provision Practice: Capturing the Dynamics of Peer Support Work in Action. *The Journal of Mental Health Training, Education and Practice 14*(2), 106–118.

Index

For Product Safety Concerns and Information please contact our EU
representative GPSR@taylorandfrancis.com
Taylor & Francis Verlag GmbH, Kaufingerstraße 24, 80331 München, Germany

www.ingramcontent.com/pod-product-compliance
Lightning Source LLC
Chambersburg PA
CBHW052001270326
41929CB00015B/2736

9 781032 714530